DIGITAL TOMOSYNTHESIS

BENEFITS, CLINICAL USES AND LIMITATIONS

BIOTECHNOLOGY IN AGRICULTURE, INDUSTRY AND MEDICINE

Additional books in this series can be found on Nova's website
under the Series tab.

Additional e-books in this series can be found on Nova's website
under the eBooks tab.

BIOTECHNOLOGY IN AGRICULTURE, INDUSTRY AND MEDICINE

DIGITAL TOMOSYNTHESIS

BENEFITS, CLINICAL USES AND LIMITATIONS

LUCIA GUTIERREZ
EDITOR

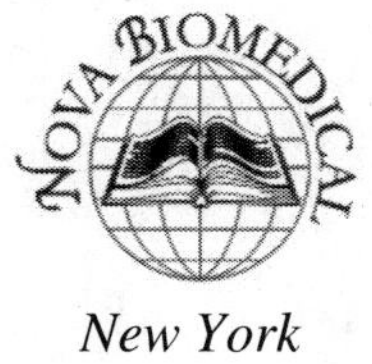

New York

NOTICE TO THE READER

Library of Congress Cataloging-in-Publication Data

Names: Gutiberrez, Lucbia M., editor.
Title: Digital tomosynthesis : benefits, clinical uses and limitations / editor, Lucia Gutierrez.
Description: Hauppauge, New York : Nova Science Publisher's, Inc., [2016] |
Series: Biotechnology in agriculture, industry and medicine | Includes index. |
Description based on print version record and CIP data provided by publisher; resource not viewed.
Identifiers: LCCN 2016018872 (print) | LCCN 2016014500 (ebook) | ISBN 9781634851466 () |
ISBN 9781634851329 (softcover) | ISBN 9781634851466 (ebook)
Subjects: LCSH: Tomosynthesis. | Breast--Radiography.
Classification: LCC RC78.7.T6 (print) | LCC RC78.7.T6 D54 2016 (ebook) | DDC 616.07/572--dc23
LC record available at https://lccn.loc.gov/2016018872

Published by Nova Science Publishers, Inc. † New York

CONTENTS

PREFACE

Tomosynthesis is a technology that enables the acquisition of three-dimensional (3D) data from a sequence of projection images acquired at different x-ray tube angles. Tomosynthesis imaging is being actively investigated for use in a variety of clinical tasks. Chapter One of this book provides a comparison of reconstruction algorithms in terms of radiation dose reduction of x-ray tomosynthesis. Digital Breast Tomosynthesis (DBT), an emerging and improving breast imaging technology, enhances the diagnosis of early breast cancer by providing in-depth information about the overlapping dense breast tissues with no ambiguities. Chapter Two reviews population-based screening/clinical trials of digital breast tomosynthesis. The last chapter discusses image reconstruction and imaging configuration optimization with a multi-beam parallel digital breast tomosynthesis system.

Chapter 1 – The authors compared reconstruction algorithms [filtered back projection (FBP), maximum likelihood expectation maximization (MLEM), and the simultaneous iterative reconstruction technique (SIRT)] in terms of radiation dose and image quality to explore the possibility of radiation dose reduction during breast and arthroplasty imaging. The three algorithms were implemented using a tomosynthesis system and experimentally evaluated the following measurements: contrast-to-noise ratio, signal difference-to-noise ratio, artifact spread function, and intensity profile. The possible radiation dose reduction, contrast improvement, and artifact reduction in tomosynthesis were evaluated using different exposure levels and the three reconstruction techniques. As MLEM and SIRT suppress streak artifacts, further investigation is required to compare these techniques to FBP. However, the advantages of each technique, such as better suppression of streak artifacts with a radiation dose reduction using MLEM and SIRT and better reproducibility using FBP, should be considered in clinical practice.

Chapter 2 – The aim of this chapter is to review the major benefits and limitations in current Digital Breast Tomosynthesis (DBT) through the population-based screening trials that are emerging. Breast cancer is the most commonly diagnosed cancer type among women and remains a leading cause of death from cancer. However, there has been a decrease of more than 36% in the death rate from breast cancer as a result of improvements in treatments and early detection. For a long time, Digital Mammography (DM) was considered as the gold standard method for breast cancer early detection but, as a two-dimensional (2D) technique, it has some crucial limitations like tissue overlapping. Nowadays, DBT has been widely referred to as a possible modality to replace DM in the screening programs. Tomosynthesis is a technology that enables the acquisition of three-dimensional (3D) data from a sequence of projection images acquired at different x-ray tube angles. Tomosynthesis imaging is being actively investigated for use in a variety of clinical tasks. Looking at PubMed database (until 2015), approximately 45% of the reported studies on tomosynthesis are related to DBT and 86% of these were published in the last five years. Based on this data it is possible to verify the current importance of DBT. Since its first demonstration in 1997, DBT has been improved and is the focus of many research in order to establish its true clinical value, especially in the screening programs. The need for this establishment and recognition have led to several large-scale screening/clinical trials. So far, there are four main trials, three of them already completed and one still in progress. The STORM trial: performed in Italy, with 7292 women. The Oslo trial: carried out in Norway, with 24901 women. The TOMMY trial: carried out in the United Kingdom, with 8869 women. And finally the one that is still in progress but already has some published results: The Malmo trial which is being performed in Sweden, with 15000 participants. This chapter reviews these population-based screening/clinical trials. Other large studies already performed will also be considered. The results from these trials can potentially provide evidence to guide the future application of DBT.

Chapter 3 – Digital breast tomosynthesis is a novel technology that provides 3D information of the breast and helps to identify the malignant cancer tissue from overlying healthy breast tissue. Optimizing image reconstruction and imaging configuration of a multi-beam parallel digital breast tomosynthesis system is in demand. Numerously used algorithms from the typical image reconstruction models which are used for iso-centric tomosynthesis systems were investigated for the present multi-beam parallel tomosynthesis imaging system. The representative algorithms, including back-projection (BP), filtered back-projection (FBP), matrix inversion tomosynthesis reconstruction (MITS), maximum likelihood expectation maximization (MLEM), ordered-subset maximum likelihood expectation maximization (OS-MLEM), and simultaneous algebraic reconstruction technique (SART), were implemented to fit our system design. Experiments, based on phantoms and computer simulations, illustrate that the prototype system combined with developed algorithms is capable of providing three-dimensional information of the objects with good image quality and has abilities to improve digital breast tomosynthesis technology. Four methodologies were employed to optimize the reconstruction algorithms and different imaging configurations were tested for the prototype system. A linear tomosynthesis imaging analysis tool was used to investigate blurring-out reconstruction algorithms. Computer simulations of sphere and wire objects were used to evaluate the performance of various out-of-plane artifact removal approaches. A frequency-domain-based methodology, relative NEQ(f) analysis, was investigated to evaluate the overall system performance based on the propagation of signal and noise. This study had three over all findings: the iterative reconstruction algorithms remove more out-of-plane blur; increasing the view angle could decrease out-of-plane blur; and increasing the number of projection images can improve the in-focus sharpness of the objects.

In: Digital Tomosynthesis
Editor: Lucia Gutierrez

ISBN: 978-1-63485-132-9
© 2016 Nova Science Publishers, Inc.

Chapter 1

X-RAY TOMOSYNTHESIS IMAGING: COMPARISON OF RECONSTRUCTION ALGORITHMS IN TERMS OF RADIATION DOSE REDUCTION

Tsutomu Gomi[*]
Kitasato University, Sagamihara, Japan

ABSTRACT

We compared reconstruction algorithms [filtered back projection (FBP), maximum likelihood expectation maximization (MLEM), and the simultaneous iterative reconstruction technique (SIRT)] in terms of radiation dose and image quality to explore the possibility of radiation dose reduction during breast and arthroplasty imaging.

The three algorithms were implemented using a tomosynthesis system and experimentally evaluated the following measurements: contrast-to-noise ratio, signal difference-to-noise ratio, artifact spread function, and intensity profile. The possible radiation dose reduction, contrast improvement, and artifact reduction in tomosynthesis were evaluated using different exposure levels and the three reconstruction techniques.

As MLEM and SIRT suppress streak artifacts, further investigation is required to compare these techniques to FBP. However, the advantages of

---

[*] gomi@kitasato-u.ac.jp.

each technique, such as better suppression of streak artifacts with a radiation dose reduction using MLEM and SIRT and better reproducibility using FBP, should be considered in clinical practice.

Keywords: tomosynthesis, radiation dose, breast, arthroplasty, wavelet denoising

INTRODUCTION

Tomosynthesis is a limited-angle image reconstruction method wherein a projection dataset of a structure acquired at regular intervals during a single acquisition pass is used to reconstruct planar sections *a priori*. Tomosynthetic slices exhibit high resolution in planes parallel to the detector plane. Furthermore, tomosynthesis provides the additional benefits of digital imaging [1-6] combined with the tomographic benefits of computed tomography (CT) at a lower radiation dose, costs less, and is easily implemented in conjunction with chest radiography. This technique was developed by improving the older geometric tomography technique that has largely fallen out of favor for chest imaging because of the positioning difficulties, high radiation doses, and residual blur caused by out-of-plane structures. Tomosynthesis has overcome these difficulties by enabling the reconstruction of numerous image slices from a single low-dose image data acquisition. Tomosynthesis images are still invariably affected by blurring because of out-of-plane structures and are superimposed on the focused fulcrum plane image by the limited acquisition angle. This can result in poor structure detectability in the in-focus plane.

To explore the possibility of decreasing the radiation dose during tomosynthesis for breast and arthroplasty imaging, we compared the image qualities of several reconstruction algorithms, such as filtered back projection (FBP) [7], and two iterative reconstruction (IR) methods: maximum likelihood expectation maximization (MLEM) [8] and simultaneous iterative reconstruction technique [SIRT (of the additive or multiplying operations, we selected the additive type in this study)] [9] under different radiation doses. The reconstruction algorithms are summarized in Figures 1–3.

Breast imaging: Digital breast tomosynthesis (DBT) is among the most promising techniques for improving early breast cancer detection. It can provide three-dimensional structural information by reconstructing an entire image volume from a sequence of projection-view mammograms acquired at a small number of projection angles over a limited angular range. The total radiation dose is comparable with that used during regular mammography screening. DBT has been shown to decrease the camouflaging effect of overlapping fibroglandular breast tissue [10], thus improving the conspicuity of subtle lesions. Several digital mammography-based DBT systems have been developed [11], and preliminary pilot clinical studies are ongoing to evaluate the utility of this technique [12-13]. Various DBT reconstruction methods have been previously explored [7, 14-15]. The recent reconstruction and image processing technique, IR and wavelet denoising processing [16] (Figure 4), was found to effectively decrease quantum noise and radiation exposure. The IR technique with wavelet denoising processing may improve the image quality and reduce the exposure dose relative to those associated with the conventional FBP technique. The two IR techniques (SIRT and MLEM) and wavelet denoising processing were evaluated and the reconstructed image qualities and possible exposure dose reductions were compared with and without wavelet denoising processing of the FBP, SIRT, and MLEM algorithms.

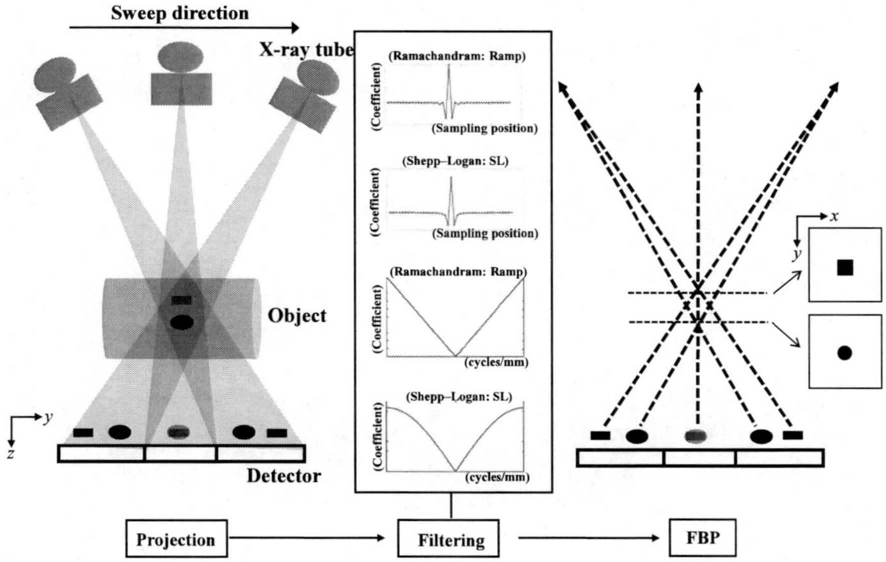

Figure 1. Concept of the filtered back projection (FBP) processing method for tomosynthesis.

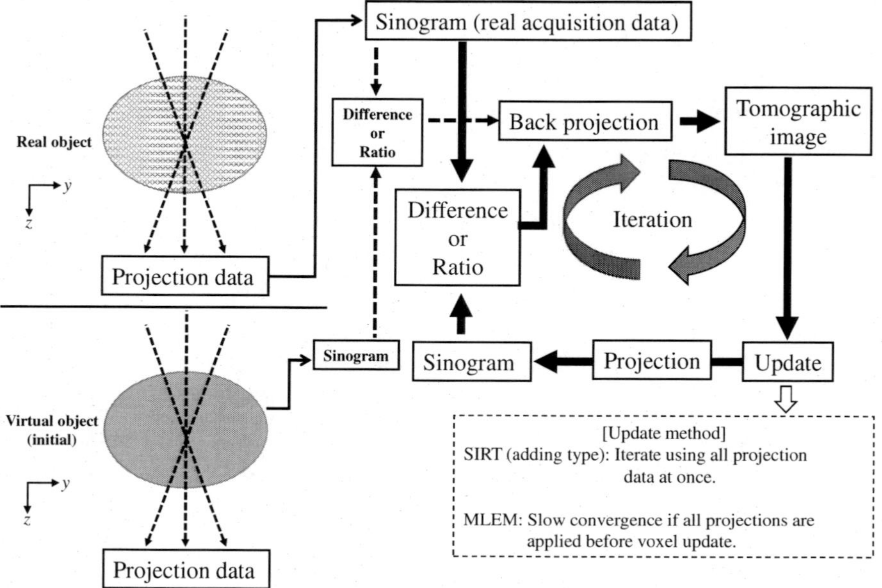

Figure 2. Concept of the iterative reconstruction (IR) processing method for tomosynthesis.

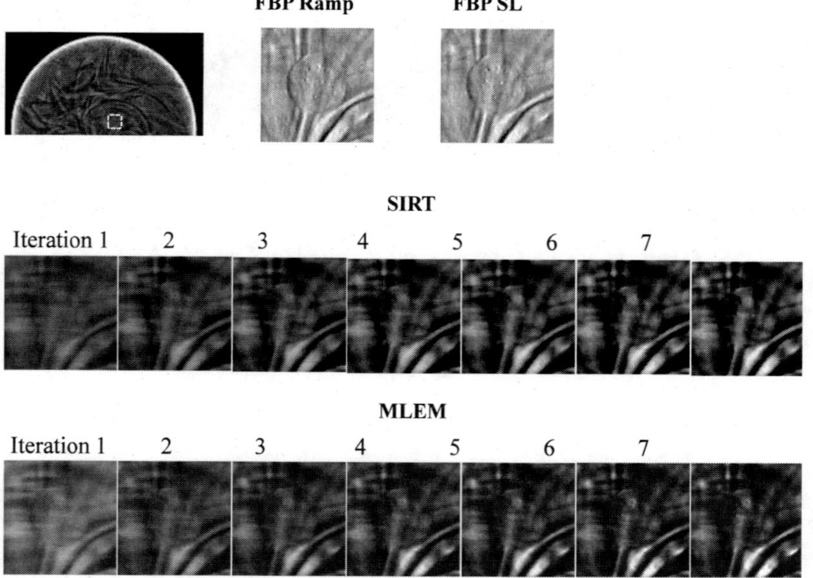

Figure 3. Iterative reconstruction (IR) reconstruction algorithm for tomosynthesis: comparison between different iteration images (BR3D phantom).

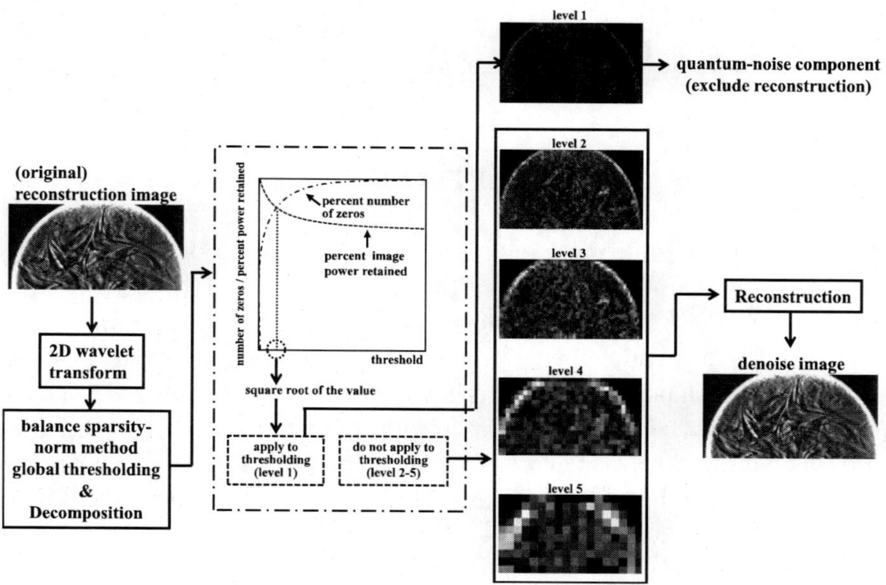

Figure 4. Wavelet denoising processing: flowchart illustrating the successive steps in the wavelet processing method.

Arthroplasty imaging: Imaging techniques provide important diagnostic information such as feature exclusion and the loosening and verification of sufficient implant coverage. Hematoma or inflammation in the adjacent soft tissue must also be assesssed. However, artifacts greatly complicate the evaluation of these features, frequently rendering the images uninterpretable by conventional image reconstructions, even when hard convolution kernels, such as FBP, are used. In digital tomosynthesis (DT), artifacts appear as very low signals along the sweep direction around the edges of highly attenuating materials such as metal prosthesis or osteosynthetic materials [17-18]. These artifacts are predominantly caused by the reconstruction of very low-level signals in the shadow of the highly attenuating object. Besides FBP, the IR method has been explored in DT for arthroplasty. IR was found to effectively decrease quantum noise and radiation exposure and may improve the image quality compared with the conventional FBP technique [19]. However, this study was limited to the comparisons of FBP, algebraic IR, and SIRT; furthermore, only a simple prosthesis and contrast detail phantom were evaluated under constant radiation doses. We evaluated and compared the characteristics of the reconstructed images and a possible radiation dose reduction by applying the conventional FBP, algebraic SIRT, and statistical MLEM algorithms to prosthesis phantoms.

METHODS

Phantom Specifications

Brest imaging: A BR3D phantom (Model 020; CIRS Inc., Norfolk, VA, USA) consists of multiple heterogeneous slabs that mimic the glandular and adipose tissue composition and parenchymal patterns of a human breast. The slabs are made of epoxy resins with X-ray attenuation properties corresponding to 50% glandular/50% adipose breast tissue. We arranged the non-target slabs at the top (20–50 mm) and bottom of the target slab (10 mm) (Figure 5).

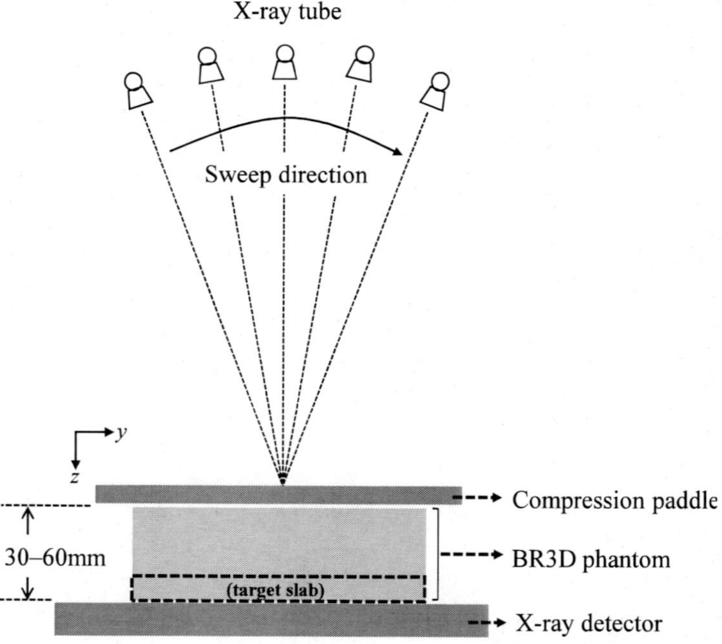

Figure 5. For digital breast tomosynthesis (DBT) acquisition, the BR3D phantom was arranged parallel to the detector plane.

Arthoroplasty imaging: To evaluate the image quality (implant and artificial bone introduced as the artifacts and contrast, respectively), we immersed a prosthesis phantom containing an implant in the center of a polymethyl methacrylate case filled with water (case dimensions: φ 200 mm × 300 mm). The area of the phantom that was filled with water was considered to a composition that simulated soft tissue because water is often used as the substitute for soft tissues in phantom experiments. The phantom was an artificial bone [Orthopedic Humerus models (Model: Normal Anatomy, canal diameter: 9 mm, overall length: 300 mm), Pacific. Research Laboratories, Inc., WA, USA]. The implant was a TRIGEN Humeral Nails Proximal Straight (Model: 38153000, diameter: 8 mm, overall length: 160 mm), from Smith & Nephew Orthopaedics KK Inc., Tokyo, Japan. In the prosthesis phantom, we assumed an internal fracture fixation (intramedullary fracture fixation) simulating a humeral proximal fracture. The prosthetic phantoms were designed to evaluate the reconstruction quality of in-focus plane and out-of-plane images (Figure 6).

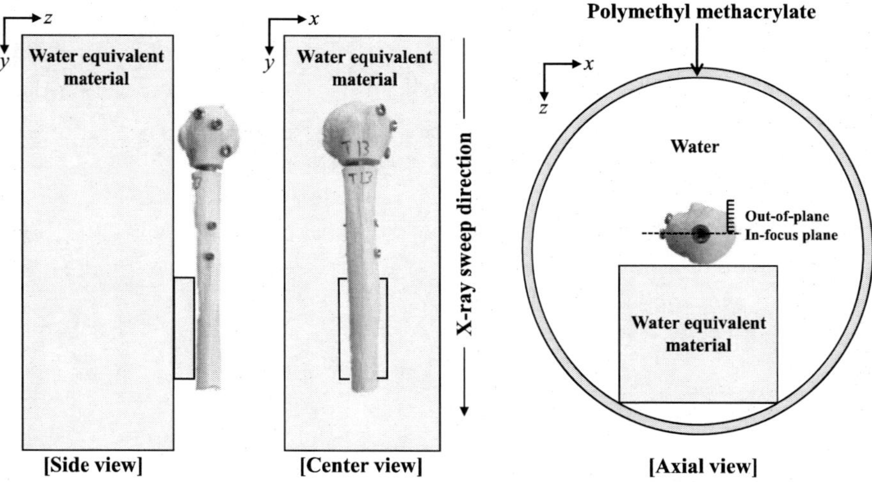

Figure 6. For digital tomosynthesis (DT) acquisition, the prosthesis phantom was arranged parallel to the detector plane.

Radiation Dose

Brest imaging: Each radiation dose setup used the following settings: a reference radiation dose [automatic exposure control (AEC) = the exposure condition at 40-mm thickness and determined tube voltage and tube current values] of 28 kVp, 50 mA; a half radiation dose of 28 kVp, 24 mA; and a quarter radiation dose of 28 kVp, 12 mA. All target and filter combinations contained tungsten (W) and rhodium (Rh). We calculated the average glandular dose (AGD) according to the method proposed by Dance et al. [20]. We used a Piranha dosimeter to measure the radiation exposure (RTI Electronics AB, Sweden). The purpose of the radiation dose measurement was to convert the established exposure condition (mA) into AGD (mGy). AGD results were as follows: for the reference radiation dose, 30-mm thickness: 1.78 mGy, 40-mm thickness: 1.51 mGy, 50-mm thickness: 1.29 mGy, and 60-mm thickness: 1.13 mGy; for the half radiation dose, 30-mm thickness: 0.93 mGy, 40-mm thickness: 0.78 mGy, 50-mm thickness: 0.67 mGy, and 60-mm thickness: 0.59 mGy; and for the quarter radiation dose, 30-mm thickness: 0.48 mGy, 40-mm thickness: 0.40 mGy, 50-mm thickness: 0.34 mGy, and 60-mm thickness: 0.30 mGy.

Arthoroplasty imaging: Tomography was performed linearly with a total acquisition time of 6.4 s [reference radiation dose: 80 kVp, 250 mA, 16 ms/view; effective dose, in accordance with the International Commission on Radiological Protection (ICRP): 0.54 mSv (ICRP 103); 20% reduced radiation dose: 80 kVp, 250 mA, 14 ms/view, 0.42 mSv; 37% reduced radiation dose: 80 kVp, 250 mA, 10 ms/view, 0.33 mSv; 55% reduced radiation dose: 80 kVp, 250 mA, 7 ms/view, 0.24 mSv]. The acquisition angle was 40°. The effective dose was calculated using the Monte Carlo-based software (PCXMC version 2.0; Radiation and Nuclear Safety Authority, Helsinki, Finland) [21]. The reference radiation dose was the dose generally used in clinical practice (the clinical task was to assess the prosthesis).

Tomosynthesis System

The DBT system (Selenia Dimensions; Hologic Inc., Bedford, MA, USA) consisted of an X-ray tube with a 0.3-mm focal spot and a digital flat-panel detector composed of amorphous selenium.

The DT system (SonialVision Safire II; Shimadzu Co., Kyoto, Japan) consisted of an X-ray tube with a 0.6-mm focal spot and digital flat-panel detector composed of amorphous selenium.

In the present study, the FBP images were reconstructed by a conventional Ramachandran-Lakshminarayanan (Ramp) or a Shepp & Logan (SL) filter kernel. In the breast imaging study, we maximized the contrast and minimized the artifacts by seven iterations of MLEM and additive SIRT. In the arthroplasty imaging study, we maximized the contrast and minimize the artifacts by 10 iterations of MLEM and additive SIRT. The FBP, MLEM, and additive SIRT image reconstruction calculations were implemented in MATLAB (Mathworks, Natick, MA, USA). The reconstruction data was real projection data acquired by a DBT and DT system. The summary of each system are shown in Tables 1 and 2.

Table 1. The detailed estimates of the digital breast tomosynthesis (DBT) acquisition parameters

Tomosynthesis system	Selenia Dimensions (Hologic Inc., Bedford, MA, USA)
Detector type	Amorphous selenium
Detector area	240 mm × 290 mm
Detector element	70 μm × 70 μm
SID*	700 mm
Target	Tungsten
Filter	Aluminum (0.7 mm)
Acquisition angle	15°
Projections	15°

Source to image distance: SID.

Table 2. The detailed estimates of the digital tomosynthesis (DT) acquisition parameters

DT system	SonialVision Safire II (Shimadzu Co., Kyoto, Japan)
Detector type	Flat-panel detector (amorphous selenium)
Detector area	362.88 mm × 362.88 mm
Detector element	150 μm × 150 μm
SID*	1100 mm
Target	Tungsten (focal spot size: 0.4 mm)
Filter	Equivalent to filtration through 3.0-mm aluminum
Acquisition angle	40°
Projections	74

Source to image distance: SID.

Evaluation

Breast Imaging

Intensity profile analysis: Different in-focus plane reconstruction methods were used to compare intensity profiles for the evaluation of the micro calcifications (0.4 mm φ; $CaCO_3$) (Figure 7).

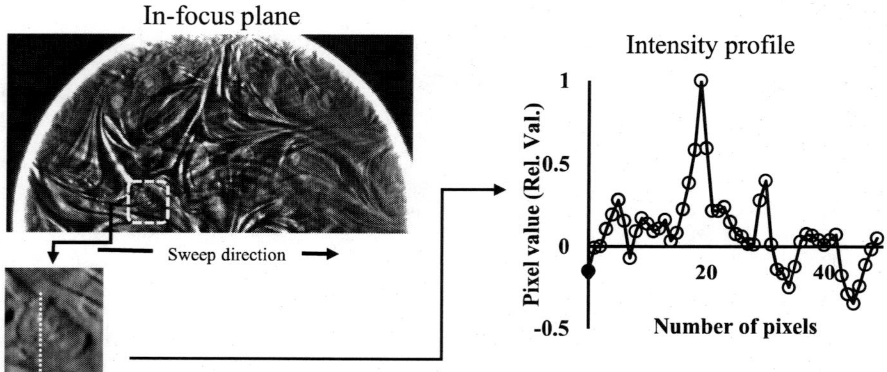

Figure 7. Areas of measurement of the intensity profile metrics (the image shown: a reconstructed image of the BR3D phantom [in-focus plane]).

Signal difference-to-noise ratio (SDNR) analysis: To quantitatively evaluate the reconstructed image quality for low-contrast resolution, we calculated the image contrast derived from SDNR [22] of selected features to determine low-contrast detectability [region of interest (ROI)-1, 6.3 mmφ; ROI-2, 4.7 mmφ; ROI1 and 2 are the same region size; spheroidal masses] at its in-focus plane for the detection of detailed bony changes. SDNR was defined as follows:

$$SDNR = |\mu_{Feature} - \mu_{BG}|/(\sigma_{Feature} - \sigma_{bg})/2 \tag{1}$$

where $\mu_{Feature}$ is the mean pixel value in the object, μ_{BG} is the mean pixel value in the background area, and $\sigma_{Feature}$ is the standard deviation of the pixel values in the background. The parameter σ_{BG} includes not only photon statistics and electronic noise in the results but also structural noise that can obscure the object (Figure 8).

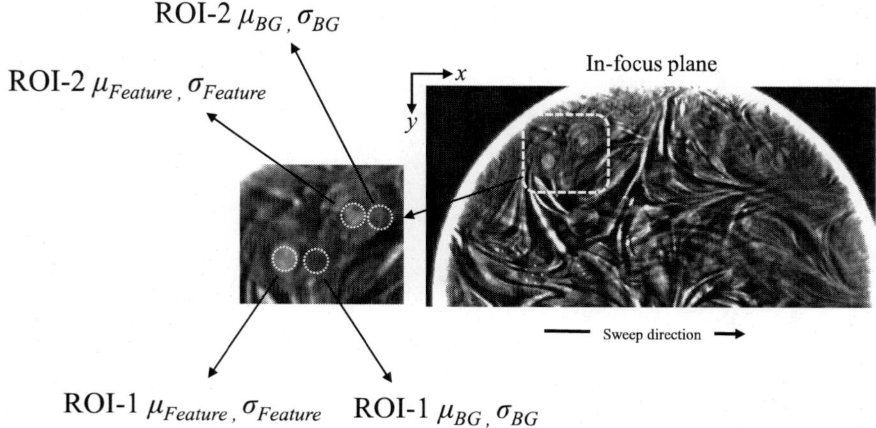

Figure 8. Areas of measurement of the signal difference-to-noise ratio (SDNR) metrics (The image shown: a reconstructed image of the BR3D phantom [in-focus plane]).

Arthoroplasty Imaging

Intensity profile analysis: We compared the intensity profiles of different reconstruction methods and radiation doses in the in-focus plane. In these comparisons, we evaluated the regions of the stem containing artifacts after processing by each technique (Figure 9).

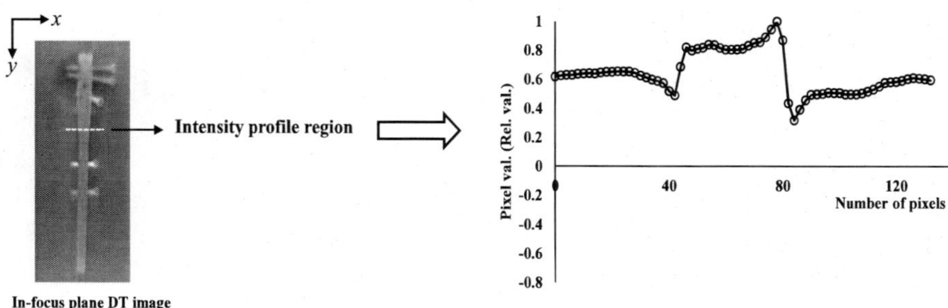

Figure 9. Areas of measurement of the intensity profile metrics (The image shown: a reconstructed image of the prosthesis phantom [in-focus plane]).

Contrast-to-noise ratio (CNR) analysis: To quantitatively evaluate the reconstructed image quality, we calculated the image contrast derived from CNR of the selected features and then determined the low-contrast detectability (34- × 14-pixel region) in the in-focus plane for the detailed detection of bone changes. CNR is defined as follows:

$$CNR = N_1 - N_0/\sigma_0 \tag{2}$$

where σ_0 is the standard deviation of the background pixel values (Figure 10).

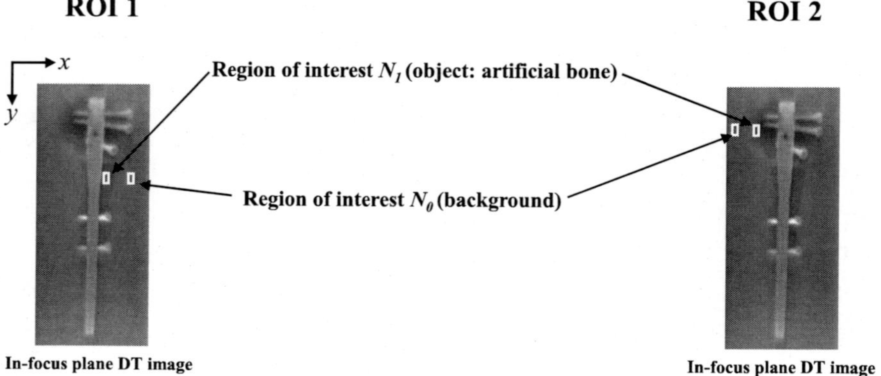

Figure 10. Areas of measurement of the contrast-to-noise ratio (CNR) metrics (The image shown: a reconstructed image of the prosthesis phantom [in-focus plane]).

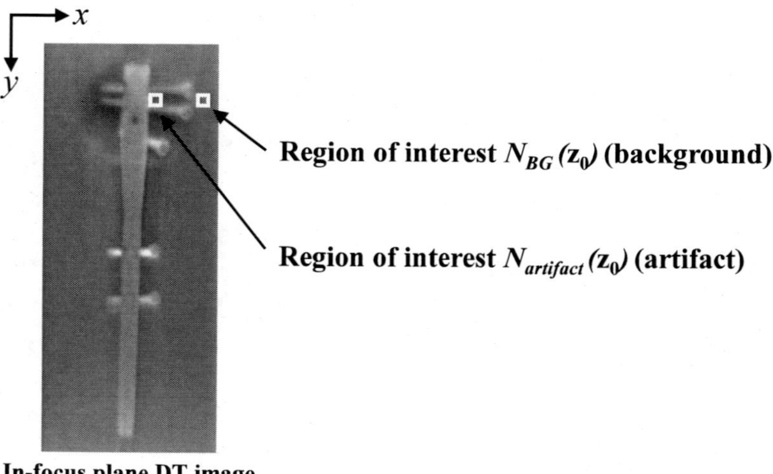

Figure 11. Areas of measurement of the artifact spared function (ASF) metrics (The image shown: a reconstructed image of the prosthesis phantom [in-focus plane]).

Artifact spread function (ASF) analysis: The ASF [23] measurement reflects the ability of DT to differentiate features that are superimposed along the tomographic slice direction. ASF of artifacts exhibited in the image plane is given as follows:

$$ASF = N_{artifact}(z) - N_{BG}(z)/N_{artifact}(z_0) - N_{BG}(z_0) \tag{3}$$

where z_0 and z are the locations of the real features in the in-focus and out-of-plane images, respectively. The ROI size in the evaluation of all features was 4 × 4 pixels (Figure 11).

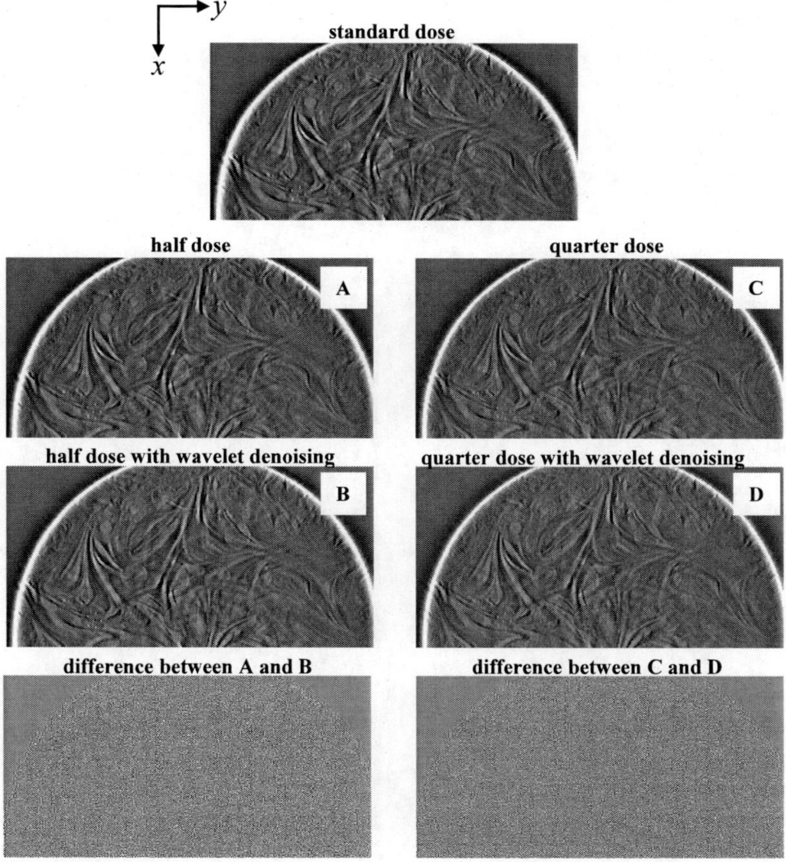

Figure 12. Comparison of the filtered back projection (FBP) reconstructed images acquired with and without wavelet processing at different exposures (x-ray sweep direction: horizontal, the image shown: a reconstructed image of the BR3D phantom [in-focus plane]).

RESULTS

Breast Imaging

The results revealed that MLEM and SIRT produced reconstructed images with features (6.3 mm φ and 4.7 mm φ, respectively) containing no artifacts in the horizontal direction (the X-ray sweep direction). Analysis of the results revealed that both DBT artifact reduction and image contrast were most effective with MLEM and SIRT at all radiation dose levels (Figures 12–14).

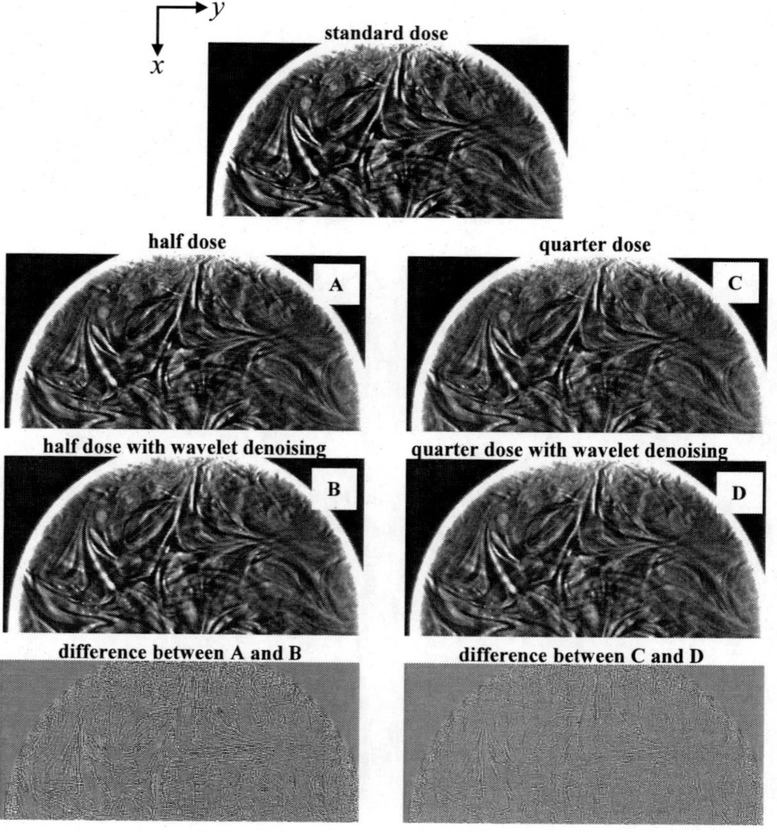

Figure 13. Comparison of the maximum likelihood expectation maximization (MLEM) reconstructed images acquired with and without wavelet processing at different exposures (x-ray sweep direction: horizontal, the image shown: a reconstructed image of the BR3D phantom [in-focus plane].

The image contrast and different diameter characteristics resulted in equivalent SDNRs (in the in-focus plane) for MLEM and SIRT. With FBP, the detectability rates for the reference radiation dose in the SDNR experiment were approximately equivalent to those of the half radiation dose images generated using MLEM and SIRT (Figure 15).

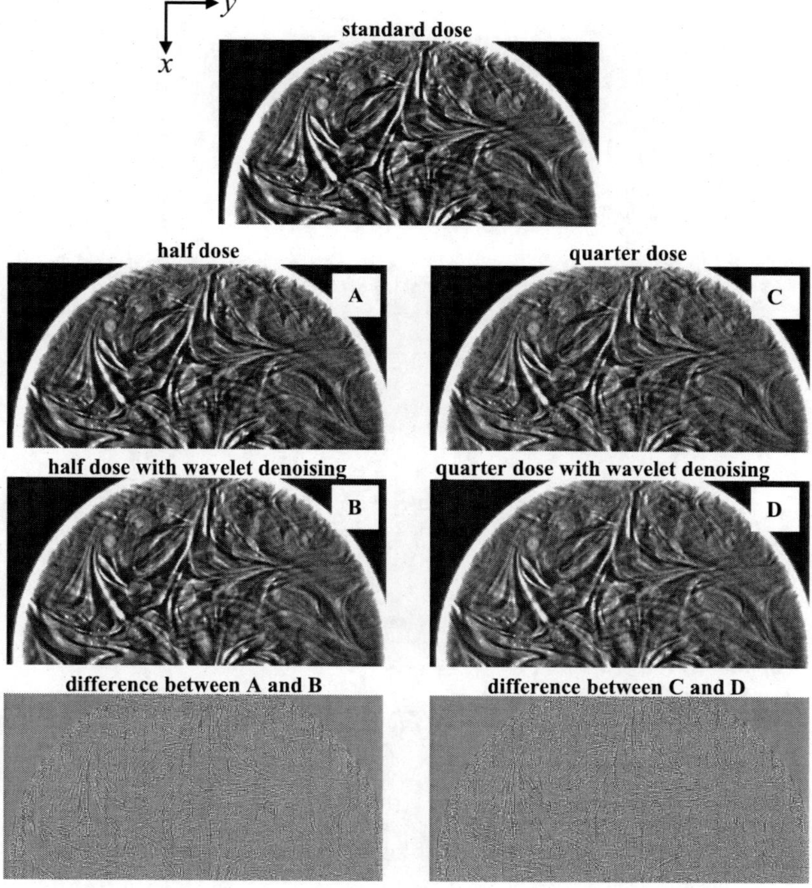

Figure 14. Comparison of the simultaneous iterative reconstruction technique (SIRT) reconstructed images acquired with and without wavelet processing at different exposures (x-ray sweep direction: horizontal, the image shown: a reconstructed image of the BR3D phantom [in-focus plane]).

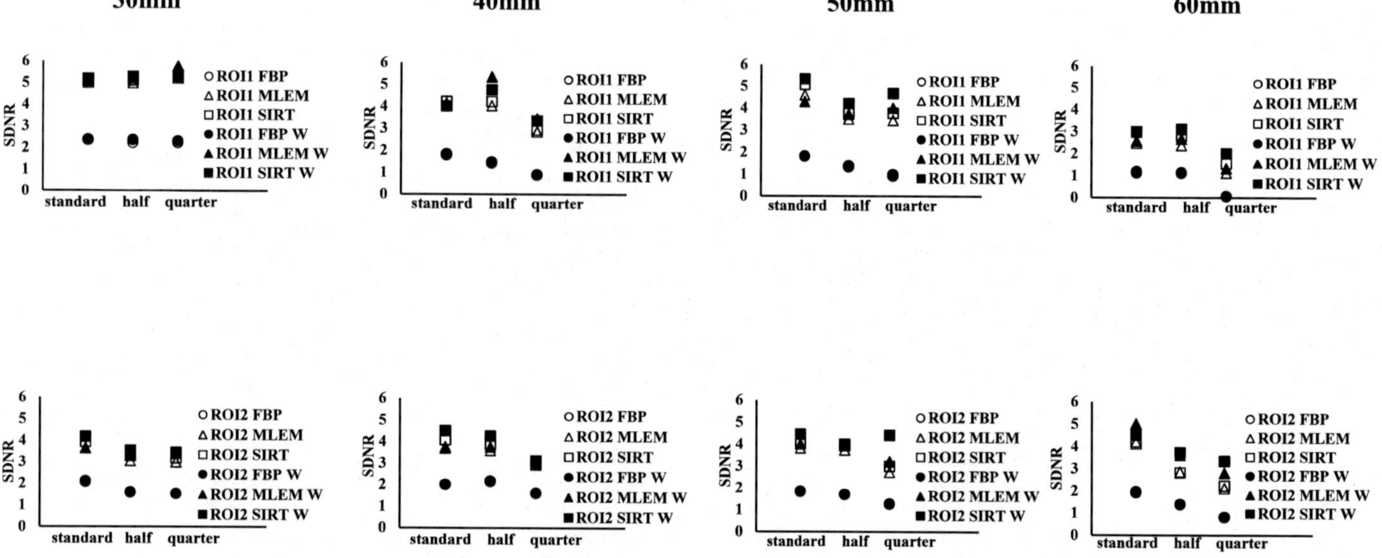

Figure 15. Comparison of the signal difference-to-noise ratio (SDNR) values obtained by using digital breast tomosynthesis (DBT) in the in-focus plane (φ 6.3 mm and φ 4.7 mm) for different phantom thicknesses and exposures. The iterative reconstruction (IR) technique was used; the contrast detectability obtained with this technique was higher than that obtained with the filtered back projection (FBP) technique.

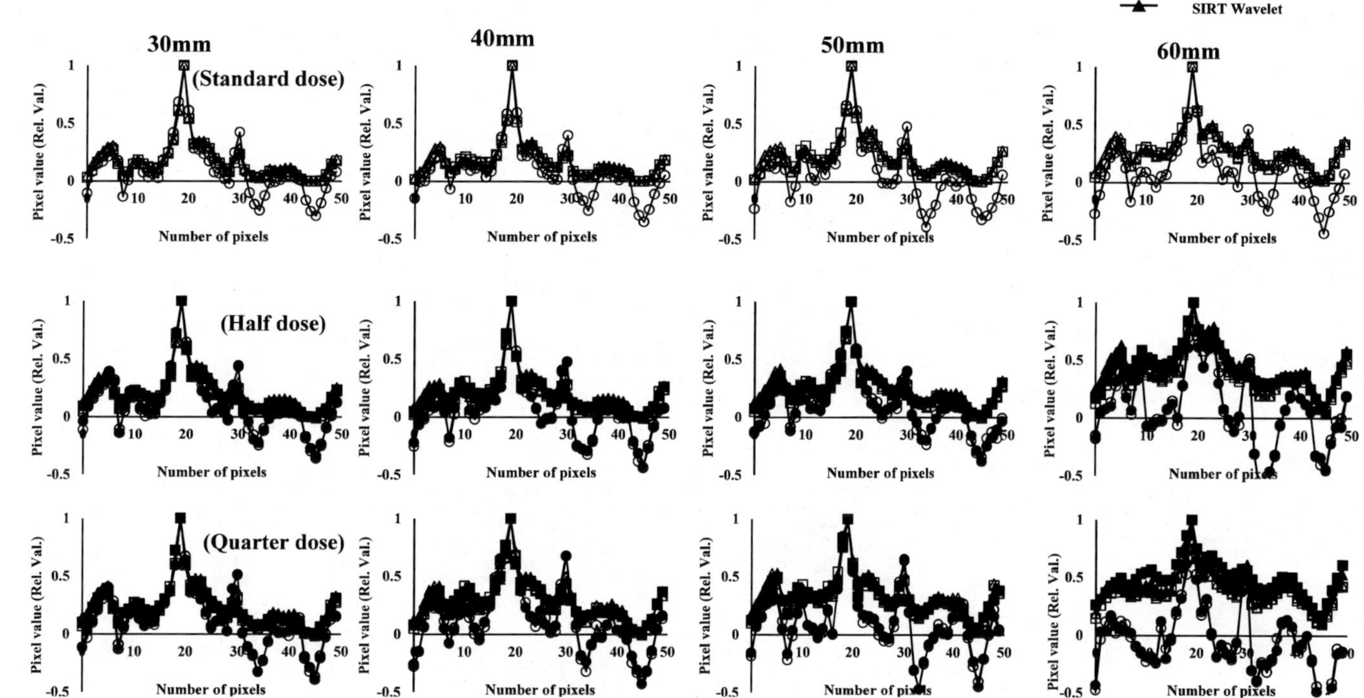

Figure 16. Comparison of the in-focus plane intensity profiles acquired using different reconstruction algorithms and different exposures [using reconstructed image of the BR3D phantom for digital breast tomosynthesis (DBT)].

Fewer artifacts were observed with MLEM and SIRT than with FBP, and the consequent improvements in image quality related to the signal undershooting were demonstrated. The intensity profiles of FBP, MLEM, and SIRT images are presented in Figure 16.

Arthoroplasty Imaging

The reconstructed images of the prosthetic phantom obtained by conventional FBP (with Ramp and SL kernels), additive SIRT, and MLEM are presented in Figure 17.

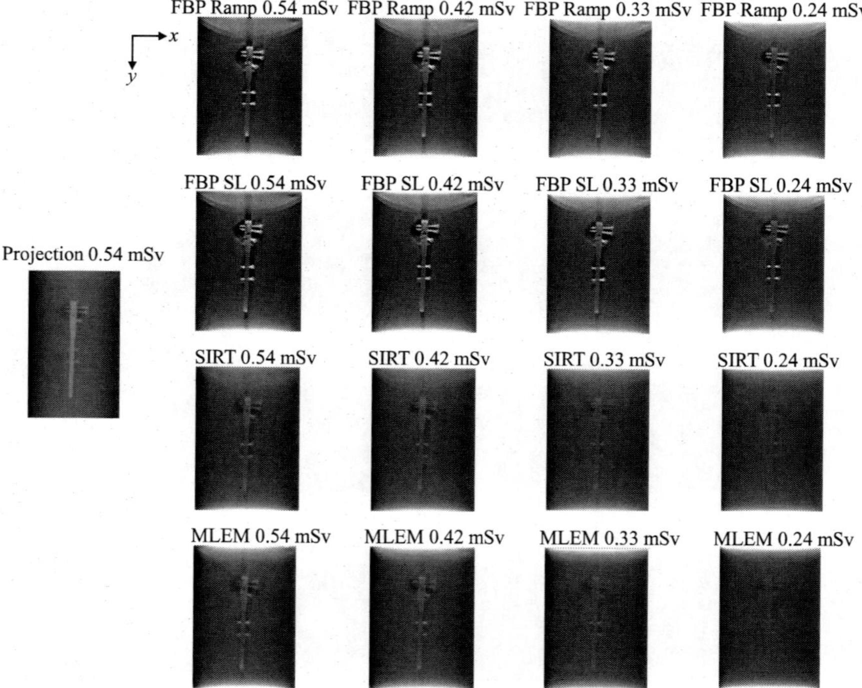

Figure 17. Comparisons between the images obtained from digital tomosynthesis (DT) and the imaging algorithms of conventional filtered back projection (FBP), simultaneous iterative reconstruction technique (SIRT), and maximum likelihood expectation maximization (MLEM) in the in-focus plane. The x-ray source is moved vertically along the image (the image shown: a reconstructed image of the prosthesis phantom).

The intensity profiles of the stem generated by the conventional FBP (with Ramp and SL kernels), additive SIRT, and MLEM are shown in Figure 18. The features in DT images generated by the additive SIRT and MLEM methods contained reduced artifacts in the vertical direction (X-ray sweep direction). In particular, artifacts were reduced in the peripheral regions of the prosthetic phantom.

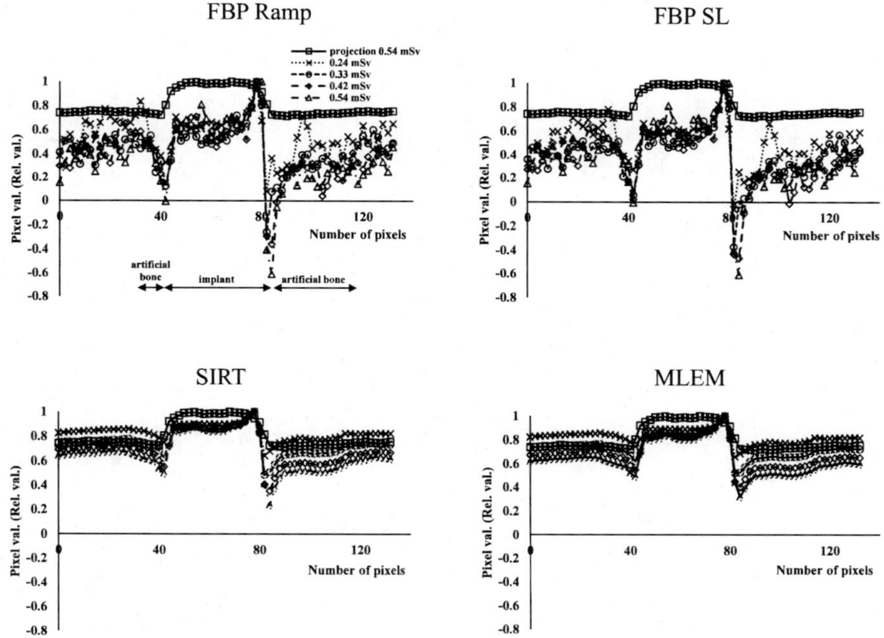

Figure 18. Comparison of the in-focus plane intensity profiles acquired using different reconstruction algorithms and different exposures [using reconstructed image of the prosthesis phantom for digital tomosynthesis (DT)].

ROIs in the prosthetic phantom experiments and plots of the CNR results are shown in Figure 19. The contrast resolution was higher in the SIRT and MLEM images than in the FBP images. The contrasts (ROI1: femoral diaphysis) in IR and FBP, the CNR difference was constant at the same radiation dose.

ROIs in the prosthetic phantom experiments and plots of the ASF results are shown in Figure 20. The additive SIRT and MLEM methods removed the highest number of artifacts. The artificial image tended to need enlargement at low radiation doses. The image quality was always superior under the reference radiation dose than under the reduced radiation doses, regardless of the method.

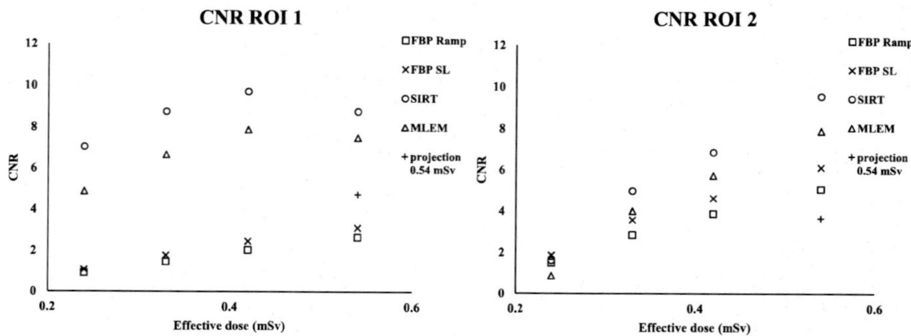

Figure 19. Comparisons of the contrast-to-noise ratios (CNR) in the in-focus plane images obtained by digital tomosynthesis (DT) under different radiation doses. Image contrast derived from the CNR of the selected two features (using reconstructed image of the prosthesis phantom).

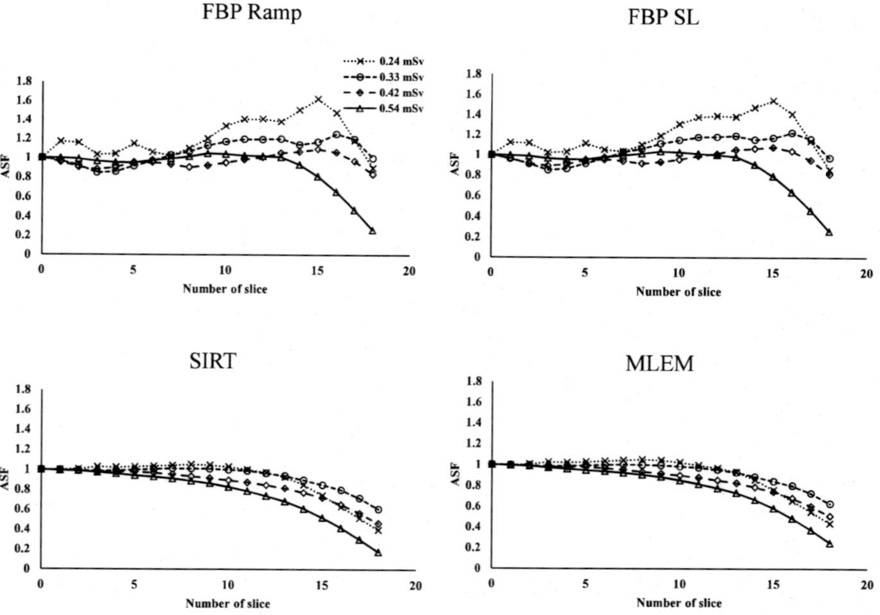

Figure 20. Plots of the artifact-spread function (ASF) versus the slice number from the in-focus plane for digital tomosynthesis (DT) images acquired under different radiation doses (using reconstructed image of the prosthesis phantom).

CONCLUSION

Breast imaging: Our experimental results clearly demonstrate that IR can be used to improve the image contrast by effectively removing quantum noise and suppressing streak artifacts in DBT images obtained using both reference and half exposure doses. Using IR, the radiation levels can be decreased to approximately half (to a 40-mm thickness) of those used for the FBP technique. In the comparison procedures with and without wavelet denoising processing, minimal improvement in the image quality with wavelet denoising processing was seen. However, there was improvement in the contrast using wavelet denoising processing for IR images at 40–50-mm thickness.

Arthoroplasty imaging: We compared various DT reconstruction methods in a prosthesis phantom study and found that the radiation levels can be decreased without largely compromising the image quality for both FBP and IR.

REFERENCES

[1]   Dobbins JT, Mcadams HP, Song JW, Li CM, Godfrey DJ, Delong DM, Paik SH, Martinez-Jimenez S., (2008). Digital tomosynthesis of the chest for lung nodule detection: interim sensitivity results from an ongoing HIH-sponsored trial. *Med. Phys.* 35, 2554-2557.

[2]   Vikgren J, Zachrisson S, Svalkvist A, Johnsson AA, Boijsen M, Flinck A, Kheddache S, Båth M., (2008). Tomosynthesis: Comparison of chest tomosynthesis and chest radiography for detection of pulmonary nodules: human observer study. *Radiology* 249, 1034-1041.

[3]   Quaia E, Baratella E, Cioffi V, Bregant P, Cernic S, Cuttin R, Cova MA., (2010). The value of digital tomosynthesis in the diagnosis of suspected pulmonary lesions on chest radiography. *Acad. Radiol.* 17, 1267-1274.

[4]   Lee G, Jeong YJ, Kim KI et al. (2013) Comparison of chest digital tomosynthesis and chest radiography for detection of asbestos-related pleuropulmonary disease. *Clin Radiol* 68: 376-382.

[5]   Sone S, Kasuga T, Sakai F, Aoki J, Izuno I, Tanizaki Y, Shigeta H, Shibata K., (1991). Development of a high-resolution digital tomosynthesis system and its clinical application. *Radiographics* 11, 807-822.

[6]   Sone S, Kasuga T, Sakai F, Kawai T, Oguchi K, Hirano H, Li F, Kudo K, Honda T, Hanouda M., (1995). Image processing in the digital tomosynthesis for pulmonary imaging. *Eur. Radiol.* 5, 96-101.

[7]   Dobbins JT 3rd, Godfrey DJ., (2003). Digital x-ray tomosynthesis: current state of the art and clinical potential. *Phys. Med. Biol.* 48, R65-106.

[8]   Wu T, Stewart A, Stanton M, McCauley T, Phillips W, Kopans DB, Moore RH, Eberhard JW, Opsahl-Ong B, Niklason L, Williams MB., (2003). Tomographic mammography using a limited number of low-dose cone-beam projection images. *Med. Phys.* 30, 365-380.

[9]   Gordon R, Bender R, Hermen GT., (1970). Algebraic reconstruction techniques (ART) for three-dimensional electron microscopy and x-ray photography. *J. Theor. Biol.* 29, 471-481.

[10] Helvie M A, Roubidoux M A, Zhang Y, Carson P L, Chan H P., (2006). Tomosynthesis mammography vs conventional mammography: lesion detection and reader reference. Initial experience. *RSNA program book*, 335.

[11] Sechopoulos I, Bliznakova K, Fei B., (2013) Power spectrum analysis of the x-ray scatter signal in mammography and breast tomosynthesis projections. *Med. Phys.* 40, 101905-1 - 101905-7.

[12] Skaane P, Bandos AI, Gullien R, Eben EB, Ekseth U, Haakenaasen U, Izadi M, Jebsen IN, Jahr G, Krager M, Niklason LT, Hofvind S, Gur D., (2013). Comparison of digital mammography alone and digital mammography plus tomosynthesis in a population-based screening program. *Radiology*, 267, 47-56.

[13] Gur D, Zuley ML, Anello MI, Rathfon GY, Chough DM, Ganott MA, Hakim CM, Wallace L, Lu A, Bandos AI., (2012). Dose reduction in digital breast tomosynthesis (DBT) screening using synthetically reconstruction projection images: an observer performance study. *Acad. Radiol.* 19, 166-171.

[14] Bleuet P, Guillemaud R, Magnin I, Desbat L., (2001). An adapted fan volume sampling scheme for 3D algebraic reconstruction in linear tomosynthesis. *IEEE. Trans. Nucl. Sci.* 3, 1720-1724.

[15] Wu T, Zhang J, Moore R, Rafferty E, Kopans D., (2004). Digital tomosynthesis mammography using a parallel maximum-likelihood reconstruction method. *Proc. SPIE.* 5368, 1-11.

[16] Gomi T, Nakajima M, Umeda T., (2015). Wavelet denoiseing for quantum noise removal in chest digital tomosynthesis. *Int. J. Comput. Assist. Radiol. Surg.* 10, 75-86.

[17] Machida H, Yuhara T, Mori T, Ueno E, Moribe Y, Sabol JM., Optimizing parameters for flat-panel detector digital tomosynthesis. *Radiographics* 30, 549-562, 2010.

[18] Gomi T, Hirano H., (2008). Clinical potential of digital linear tomosynthesis imaging of total joint arthroplasty. *J. Digit. Imaging* 21, 312-322.

[19] Gomi T., (2013). Comparison of metal artifact in digital tomosynthesis and computed tomography for evaluation of phantoms. *J. Biomed. Sci. Eng.* 6, 722-731, 2013.

[20] Dance D R, Young K C, van Engen R E., (2011). Estimation of mean glandular dose for breast tomosynthesis: factors for use with the UK, European and IAEA breast dosimetry protocols. *Phys. Med. Biol.* 56, 453-471.

[21] Tapiovaara M, Siiskonen T., (2008). A Monte Carlo program for calculating patient doses in medical x-ray examinations (2nd Ed.). Report No. STUK-A231 STUK, Helsinki, Finland.

[22] Li K, Ge Y, Garrett J, Bevins N, Zambelli J, Chen GH., (2014). Grating-based phase contrast tomosynthesis imaging: proof-of-concept experimental studies. *Med. Phys.* 41, 011903-1 – 011903-11.

In: Digital Tomosynthesis
Editor: Lucia Gutierrez

ISBN: 978-1-63485-132-9
© 2016 Nova Science Publishers, Inc.

Chapter 2

DIGITAL BREAST TOMOSYNTHESIS: A REVIEW OF POPULATION-BASED SCREENING/CLINICAL TRIALS

Ana M. Mota, Pedro Almeida and Nuno Matela*
Universidade de Lisboa, Faculdade de Ciências,
Instituto de Biofísica e Engenharia Biomédica, Lisboa, Portugal

ABSTRACT

The aim of this chapter is to review the major benefits and limitations in current Digital Breast Tomosynthesis (DBT) through the population-based screening trials that are emerging.

Breast cancer is the most commonly diagnosed cancer type among women and remains a leading cause of death from cancer. However, there has been a decrease of more than 36% in the death rate from breast cancer as a result of improvements in treatments and early detection.

For a long time, Digital Mammography (DM) was considered as the gold standard method for breast cancer early detection but, as a two-dimensional (2D) technique, it has some crucial limitations like tissue overlapping. Nowadays, DBT has been widely referred to as a possible modality to replace DM in the screening programs.

Tomosynthesis is a technology that enables the acquisition of three-dimensional (3D) data from a sequence of projection images acquired at different x-ray tube angles. Tomosynthesis imaging is being actively

---

* Corresponding author: Email: ammota@fc.ul.pt.

investigated for use in a variety of clinical tasks. Looking at PubMed database (until 2015), approximately 45% of the reported studies on tomosynthesis are related to DBT and 86% of these were published in the last five years. Based on this data it is possible to verify the current importance of DBT.

Since its first demonstration in 1997, DBT has been improved and is the focus of many research in order to establish its true clinical value, especially in the screening programs. The need for this establishment and recognition have led to several large-scale screening/clinical trials.

So far, there are four main trials, three of them already completed and one still in progress. The STORM trial: performed in Italy, with 7292 women. The Oslo trial: carried out in Norway, with 24901 women. The TOMMY trial: carried out in the United Kingdom, with 8869 women. And finally the one that is still in progress but already has some published results: The Malmo trial which is being performed in Sweden, with 15000 participants.

This chapter reviews these population-based screening/clinical trials. Other large studies already performed will also be considered. The results from these trials can potentially provide evidence to guide the future application of DBT.

Keywords: breast cancer, breast cancer screening, digital breast tomosynthesis

INTRODUCTION

Cancer is a major public health problem worldwide and is the second leading cause of death after cardiovascular diseases [1, 2]. In the United States of America (USA), breast cancer is the most commonly diagnosed cancer in women, expecting to account for 29% all new cancer diagnoses in 2016. It represents the second most common cause of cancer death in women (14%) being only surpassed by lung and bronchus cancer (26%) [3].

In the last two decades, there has been a decrease of 36% in cancer death rate from this disease as a result of improvements in early detection and treatment [3, 4]. For a long time, mammography was considered as the gold standard method for breast cancer early detection in screening programs. However, mammography generates two-dimensional (2D) images of a three-dimensional (3D) object, resulting in tissue superposition and often creating the need for unnecessary second examinations or biopsies, with additional dose, costs and anxiety for patients [5, 6].

Digital Breast Tomosynthesis (DBT) is a technique which allows to create a volumetric image of breast tissue, improving the perception of lesions' location and shape in space, without increasing the radiation dose to the patient, relative to the mammography [7]. DBT has the potential to reduce or eliminate mammography limitations and, therefore, has been widely referred to as a possible modality to replace it in the screening programs [8-10]. Yet, its true clinical value, especially in the screening programs, still need to be established and recognized. For this reason, in the last five years, there has been an increasing number of published studies, including the first large-scale screening/clinical trials.

This chapter begins by describing the main aspects about breast cancer, breast imaging in general and DBT in particular and then delves into largest studies and trials already published about the role of DBT in screening and clinical practice.

BREAST CANCER

It is believed that the first reference to cancer (not called by this name) dates back to about 3000 BC and was taken in Egypt. Later, in 460-370 BC, Hippocrates used the Greek terms *carcinos* and *carcinoma* to describe this disease and, in 28-50 BC, the Roman physician Celsus translated the Greek term into the Latin word "cancer" [1, 11].

The word "cancer" is used to identify more than 100 different and distinct diseases. These diseases all have a common point: division and uncontrolled growth of cells. Generally, these cells result from normal cells that have suffered irreparable damage of deoxyribonucleic acid (DNA). This set of cells is named as tumor. Tumors can be benign or malignant and the first are usually more controlled and not life threatening. On the other side, in a malignant tumor (or cancer), cells tend to proliferate in an uncontrolled way and, in some cases, to metastasize. When this happens, the cancer cells travel to other parts of the body through the bloodstream or lymphatic vessels [1]. The name given to most cancers arises from the primary tumor. For example, when we refer to breast cancer, we are talking about a cancer whose initial tumor was originated in the breast, even if it spreads to other parts of the body.

In 2012, cancers figure among the leading causes of morbidity and mortality worldwide, with approximately 14.000.000 new cases (more than half of these occurred in economically developing countries) and 8.200.000 cancer related deaths. The number of new cases is expected to rise to about

21.700.000 over the next two decades and, by then, 13.000.000 cancer deaths are predicted. Worldwide, the two most common cancers diagnosed in 2012 were lung (1.241.600) and prostate cancer (1.111.700) in men; and breast (1.676.600) and colorectum cancer (614.300) in women. In 2012, the estimated number of breast cancer deaths in women worldwide was 521.900 [2, 12].

In the USA (considered as one reference to a developed country) the overall estimates for 2016 are: 1.685.210 new cancer cases and 595.690 cancer deaths. For women, the two most commonly diagnosed cancers are breast (246.660, 29%) and lung & bronchus (106.470, 13%). On the other hand, the most common causes of cancer death are due to the lung & bronchus (72.160, 26%) and breast cancer (40.450, 14%). When women aged 20 to 59 years are considered, breast cancer is the leading cause of cancer death. Even though less common, breast cancer can also be diagnosed in men (2.600 estimated new cases in 2016) [3].

Over the past two decades, the increase in breast cancer incidence in women results from changes in female reproductive patterns and the increased detection of asymptomatic disease during the mammography screening [13]. Simultaneously, the decline in breast cancer death rates (about 36%) is driven by improvements in early detection and treatment [3].

Early diagnosis of breast cancer is considered vital. It is known that a 5-year relative survival rate varies from 100% for stages 0 and I (early stages) to 22% for stage IV [14]. This early detection can be performed essential by breast self-examinations, clinical breast examinations and breast imaging technology [15]. The first two methods showed no improvement in breast cancer mortality rates [16] and, very often, due to the lack of typical symptoms and signs, early-stage breast cancer is only found during breast cancer screening with imaging technology.

BREAST CANCER IMAGING

Besides the imaging modalities described below, there are many other under investigation, such as: scintimammography, single-photon emission mammography, diffraction techniques, Raman spectroscopy, optical imaging, electrical impedance spectroscopy, microwave imaging and thermography [15].

2D Mammography

Between late 1950s and early 1970s, the first results that confirmed the potential of mammography for breast cancer screening were reported [17]. The first completely dedicated mammography unit was developed in France in the middle 1960s [18] and it is currently the most widely used imaging modality for breast cancer screening. Several large randomized clinical trials have shown that mammography reduces mortality from breast cancer [19-24].

With breast under compression, it uses low-dose x-rays to acquire 2D images of the breast tissue. These images can be captured on film (screen-film mammography) or stored directly onto a computer (Digital Mammography - DM).

Screen-film mammography was one of the first technologies introduced in breast imaging and it has been the standard for detecting breast cancer for more than 30 years [15]. It has the ability to provide adequate visualization of soft tissue abnormalities, as well as depict subtle calcifications. Nevertheless, it also presents several limitations such as limited dynamic range, contrast resolution and granularity. Some studies reported the sensitivity and specificity ranges for screen-film mammography to be 62-66% and 92-98%, respectively [25-27]. It is important to keep in mind that these values are affected by breast density [28].

Since its approval by Food and Drug Administration (FDA) in 2000 [29], DM has rapidly replaced screen-film mammography as the modality of choice for screening and diagnosis of breast cancer. It overcomes several technical limitations associated with screen-film mammography, but the most significant property is that it decouples the process of image acquisition from the subsequent stages of archiving, retrieval and image display. In screen-film mammography these processes are all linked [30]. The equipment are 10 to 40 times more expensive to buy but yield cost savings by removing the films, the chemicals and by reducing the need to recall patients due to poor image quality. Once again, sensitivity and specificity depend on breast density, but the overall values are about to 70-77% and 92-97%, respectively [26, 27].

Mammography generates 2D images of a 3D object resulting in tissue superposition. This represents a key problem because it can lead to hidden malignancies and/or normal tissue considered to be pathological [8], often creating the need for unnecessary second examinations or biopsies, with additional costs and anxiety for patients [5, 6].

An example of a screen-film mammogram and a digital mammogram is presented in Figure 1.

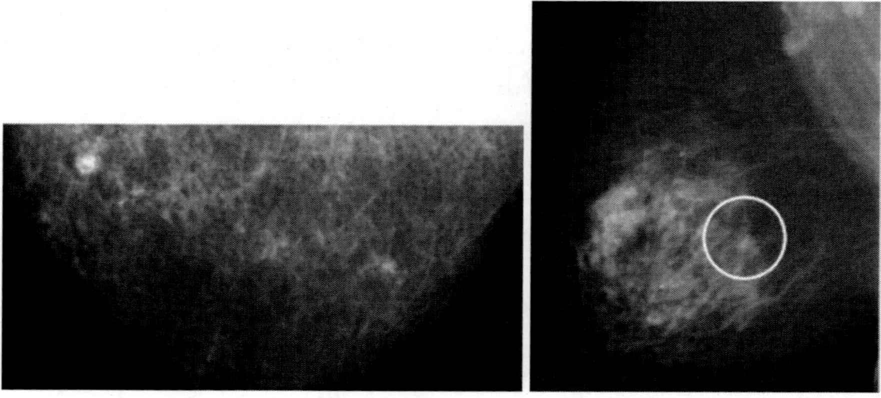

Figure 1. Example of a screen-film mammogram (left) and a digital mammogram (right) [31, 32].

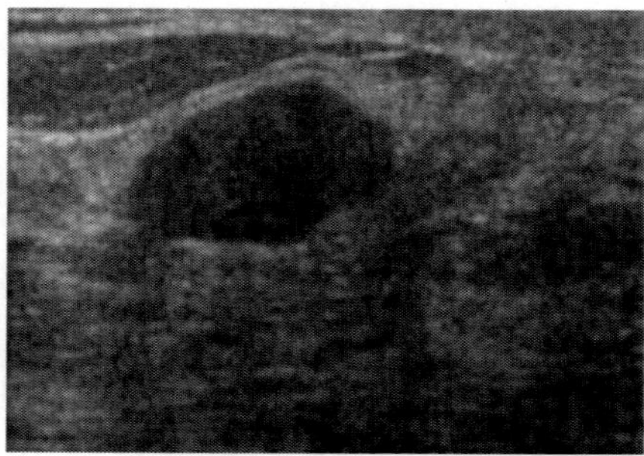

Figure 2. Example of a breast-US image [40].

Breast Ultrasound

Breast-ultrasound (US) imaging involves the use of a small transducer placed on the breast surface that transmitted high-frequency sound waves (typically 10 MHz) into the breast tissue. Then, it collects the reflected waves and use them to create continuous real-time images. US examinations are non-invasive and do not use ionizing radiation (such as x-rays). Breast-US have a greater ability than mammography to differentiate among types of normal tissues and to characterize complex cysts and solid nodules [33]. In fact, in conjunction with mammography, it may increase the accuracy of cancer detection by 50% because, in addition to the mentioned advantages, it is also very useful for dense breast evaluations [34-36]. However, one of the major drawback of breast-US as screening modality is the high number of false-negative and false-positive findings [34, 37]. The latter lead to more procedures (including biopsies) that in 70-90% of cases correspond to benign lesions [38, 39].

An example of a breast ultrasound image is presented in Figure 2.

Breast Magnetic Resonance Imaging

Breast-Magnetic Resonance Imaging (MRI) uses a powerful magnetic field and radio frequency waves pulses to change the alignment of hydrogen nuclei and thus create high contrast images of breast tissue. It is possible since hydrogen nuclei is abundant in water and fat and, these, are abundant in breast tissue. The development of a bilateral breast coil which enables simultaneous imaging of both breasts was an important technological advance [18, 41, 42]. Nowadays, a gadolinium-based contrast agent is commonly used in contrast enhanced breast MRI [43-45].

Breast-MRI is a widely used imaging modality as an adjunctive tool for screening and as a diagnostic tool for breast cancer. The sensitivity of breast-MRI in visualizing invasive cancer is nearly 100% [43] and some previous studies have showed that breast-MRI has higher sensitivity than 2D mammography [46]. Therefore, breast-MRI is an attractive option in the younger high-risk woman due to its potential to evaluate breasts in which density may limit the sensitivity of a mammogram.

Currently, breast-MRI also helps to provide information about vascular changes associated with angiogenesis[47] and is now being used to assess tumor response to treatments [48].

However, as a screening tool, MRI presents some weaknesses, such as: a significant false-positive rate, lower specificity values in comparison with 2D mammography [49], its questionable ability to detect ductal carcinoma in situ (DCIS) [44], it is slow (30 min to one hour), it may not show all calcifications [50] and the high cost [51]. Despite these main limitations, there are others that should also be considered, such as the inability to perform breast-MRI in particular patient cohorts, including those suffering from claustrophobia and individuals with metallic implants.

An example of a breast-MRI image of both breasts is presented in Figure 3.

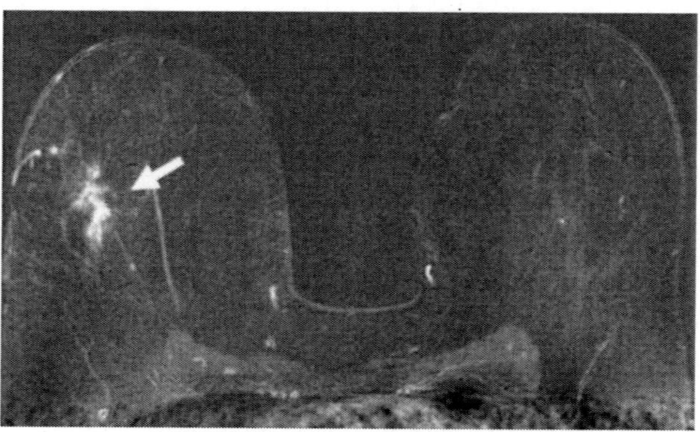

Figure 3. Example of a breast-MRI image of both breasts [42].

Positron Emission Mammography

Positron emission tomography (PET) is a nuclear medicine imaging modality used to observe metabolic processes in the body. A PET scan is useful in revealing or evaluating several conditions including cancers, heart disease and brain disorders. A radiotracer, compound by a molecule which is glucose analog labeled by a positron-emitting radioactive isotope, is injected into the patient. Malignant cells are characterized by increased glucose metabolism compared with normal cells. Therefore, the PET system detects a pair of gamma rays which are emitted from the radioisotope near the cancer cells, producing a good contrast between cancerous and normal cells. In this way, PET images provide unique functional information and can play an important role in early cancer detection through detection of residual active disease (not yet suffered anatomical changes, for example).

However, in whole body PET, spatial resolution is not sufficient for imaging early stage breast cancer [52]. In 1994, in order to overcome the limited sensitivity and spatial resolution of whole-body PET systems, the first dedicated positron emission mammography (PEM) system was developed [53]. Since then, several other systems that offer the potential of improved resolution and sensitivity have been developed [54-60].

When compared to PET and MRI, PEM showed sensitivity values from 85% to 93% for unsuspected lesions and known index lesions, respectively [61]. In fact, PEM and breast-MRI are very similar about the sensitivity and specificity values, with values of 92-97% for PEM [62]. Despite the satisfying values shown about sensitivity and specificity, PEM has a major limitation:

radiation exposure. In terms of relative risk to a 40-year-old woman, in a single PEM study (involving the use of a label-recommended radioisotope), the dose is associated with a 15 times higher risk of cancer induction than a single screen-film or digital mammogram. In PEM, all body organs are irradiated with radioisotopes, so it can lead to cancer induction not only in the breast (such as mammography) but also in any other radiosensitive organ [61]. This is one of the main reasons PEM is not considered as a screening modality. However, with continued advancement of detector technology, PEM are likely to play a significant role in therapeutic monitoring of known cancers and in diagnostic imaging of suspicious breast lesions [18].

An example of a PEM image is presented in Figure 4.

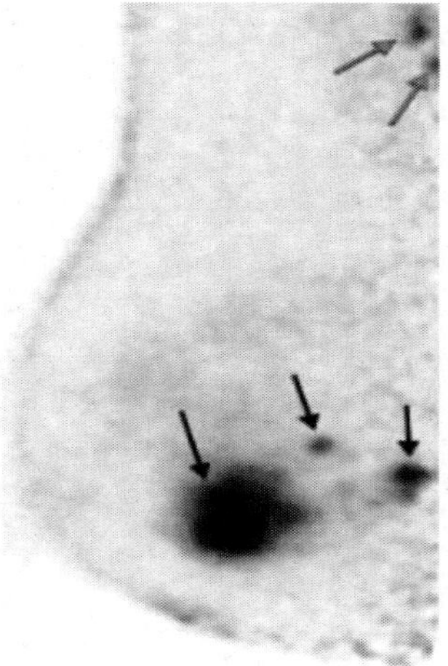

Figure 4. Example of a PEM image [61].

Breast Computed Tomography

Dedicated breast-computed tomography (CT) represents a new x-ray technology which may allow true 3D imaging generated from a large series of 2D images or slices. Breast-CT offers some advantages over other modalities, such as: it does not require physical compression of the breast as mammography, greatly alleviating patient discomfort; and its images do not experience the distortion seen in MRI and so regular biopsy needles can be used [63].

An initial study, comparing non-contrast breast-CT with screen-film mammography, showed that overall conspicuity of breast lesions on breast-CT was equal to that on 2D mammography. In fact, it suggests that breast-CT was superior for visualization of masses but was inferior for visualization of microcalcifications [31]. Another study, with an intravenous contrast agent, was performed in order to evaluate lesion conspicuity on contrast enhanced breast-CT images and on 2D mammograms [64]. It revealed that the use of intravenous contrast in breast-CT enhances the visualization of malignant lesions, including microcalcifications.

The need to use a contrast agent for a reasonable visualization of microcalcifications imposes a drawback to this technique, since the group of people who can benefit from it decreases. Therefore, the poor visualization of microcalcifications on unenhanced breast-CT means a significant limitation to the use of this modality for breast cancer screening in the general population. Nevertheless, breast-CT may play an important role in breast cancer imaging.

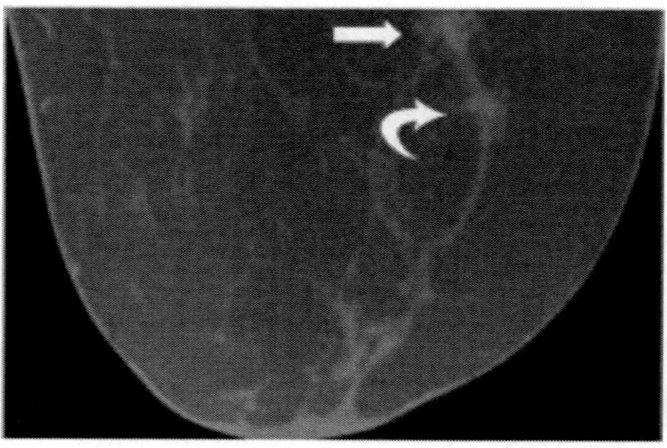

Figure 5. Example of a breast-CT image [31].

Additionally, there are some other challenging points in order to adopt breast-CT in clinical practice such as: to coverage the entire breast, including the axillary tail extending to the chest wall [65]; the need for the subject to remain still, while holding their breath for the duration of the scan (~9-second scan) [63]; and the expected cost that should be more reasonable than MRI but still much more expensive than mammography [65].

The development of breast-CT is at an early stage. Current systems used in clinical studies [31, 63, 66, 67] are prototypes and further clinical comparison of breast-CT with other established modalities is required in order to determine its optimal and most cost-effective application strategy.

An example of a breast-CT image is presented in Figure 5.

DIGITAL BREAST TOMOSYNTHESIS

Development of Digital Breast Tomosynthesis

Digital tomosynthesis imaging is a quasi-3D x-ray imaging modality in which slice images are reconstructed from a series of projections acquired from a limited angle x-ray scan. Tomosynthesis introduces depth information with little or no increase in radiation dose when compared to conventional x-ray imaging. In this way, it addresses one of the primary weaknesses of conventional x-ray imaging: the superposition of objects in the image. This superposition may result in hidden object of interest and/or mimic disease. By generating slice images, tomosynthesis is able to decrease superposition [68, 69].

The first reference to this technique was done in 1935 through the name "seriescopy" [70]. The word "tomosynthesis" was used for the first time by Grant in 1972 [71]. There were almost no developments in tomosynthesis until the late 1990s. The renewed interest began with the new generation of flat-panel detectors, the application of tomosynthesis to full-field and small field breast imaging [72, 73] and the application of tomosynthesis to chest imaging [74].

Looking at PubMed database (until 2015), for "Tomosynthesis [Title/Abstract]" 810 publications were identified, the first of which corresponds to the first time the word was mentioned (1972) [71]. Over the past 10 years, there has been a significant increase in the number of publications: from 7 in 2005 to 151 in 2015 (about 22 times more). For "Breast Tomosynthesis [Title/Abstract]," 369 publications were found. The current importance of digital breast tomosynthesis (DBT) is confirmed by two facts: 45% of the reported studies on tomosynthesis are related to DBT and 86% of these studies were published in the last five years. The progress of the number of publications about "tomosynthesis" and "breast tomosynthesis" is well presented in Figure 6.

DBT had received approval for clinical use in Europe and Canada in 2008 and FDA approval in the USA in 2011. Therefore, in addition to PubMed results, we can state that, currently, DBT imaging is at the forefront.

The overlying fibroglandular tissue in the image is referred as one of the main shortcoming of mammography. In the case of breast cancer detection, dense fibroglandular tissue may obscure mammographic signs of malignancy resulting in hidden or "missed" cancers. On the other hand, fibroglandular tissue may superimpose to falsely mimic a mammographic abnormality leading to an unnecessary recall for additional imaging DBT has the potential to reduce or eliminate these limitations. It allows to create tomographic images of a tissue volume, improving the perception of lesions' location and shape in space, without increasing the radiation dose to the patient, relative to conventional DM [7]. On the other hand, an important benefit of DBT is that it has an acquisition geometry very similar to conventional mammography. Therefore, it may be easy to implement and adapt in clinical practice.

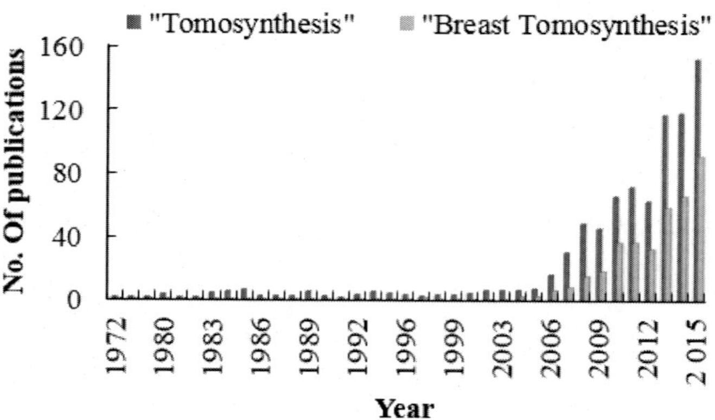

Figure 6. Number of publications per year (until 2015) for "Tomosynthesis [Title/Abstract]" and "Breast Tomosynthesis [Title/Abstract]" in PubMed database.

Table 1. Design specifications for several DBT systems [29, 69, 87-89]

	GE Senoclaire	Hologic Selenia Dimensions	IMS Giotto Tomo	Philips (Sectra)	Siemens Mammomat Inspiration
Scan angle (°)	25	15	40	11	50
No. Of projections	9	15	13	21	25
Acquisition time (secs)	7	4	12	3-10	25
Tube motion	Step & shoot	Continuous	Continuous	Continuous	Continuous
Detector Motion	No	Yes	No	Yes	No
Detector	CsI/a-Si	a-Se	a-Se	Silicon	a-Se
Pixel pitch (μm)	100	70	85	50	85
Reconstruction	Iterative	FBP	Iterative	Iterative	FBP
FDA approval	2014	2011	-	-	2015

CsI/a-Si: Cesium Iodide/amorphous Silicon.
a-Se: Amorphous Selenium FBP: Filtered Back Projection.

Optimization of acquisition parameters for breast tomosynthesis continues to be an area of considerable research [75-86]. In addition to breast imaging, chest tomosynthesis and detection of hairline fractures with tomosynthesis skeletal imaging are also being investigated [69].

System Designs

DBT systems from different manufacturers vary in their specifications and only a few have received FDA approval. Table 1 demonstrates some of the design differences of those breast imaging systems.

Advantages and Disadvantages of DBT

A brief summary of the potential advantages and disadvantages of DBT is presented in Table 2 [15, 89-92].

Advances in DBT

Lesions presenting architectural distortion are particularly difficult to localize by breast-US (sometimes leading to false negative needle biopsies) and to visualize with 2D mammographic views (cannot be targeted using traditional stereotactic vacuum-assisted biopsy techniques guided by 2D mammography). Currently, these cases are referred to breast-MRI performed with MR-guided vacuum-assisted biopsy. However, this leads to delays in patient care, as well as increased radiological costs and extra stress for the patients [93]. DBT guided biopsy systems are referred as being particularly useful in such cases because these lesions are usually well visualized with DBT. In addition, these systems allow faster lesion targeting, fewer x-ray exposures and reduced patient procedure time [94, 95].

DBT has a higher number of images to review, so it does take longer to interpret and this may impose clinical workflow challenges. Besides, physician oversight of findings could increase. Therefore, DBT computer-assisted detection (CAD) could play a significant role in improving workflow efficiency and may have a more significant clinical role than with conventional DM in improving work performance. Currently, CAD is available for clinical applications for 2D imaging and, although current DM CAD algorithms cannot be directly applied to DBT image data, there is active research in this field [96-100]. In fact, data suggest that CAD could perform better with DBT images compared to DM images. It is possible because, with DBT, the margins of masses and subtle areas of distortion are better depicted which could lead to more true-positive CAD marks. Hence, the DBT CAD system is a viable tool that could help in the efficiency of DBT image interpretation [90].

Table 2. Summary of some advantages and disadvantages of DBT imaging

Advantages	Disadvantages
(1) DBT systems only require minor alterations to existing mammographic systems. (2) DBT systems are able to take conventional mammograms as well. (3) DBT imaging helps in the detection of architectural distortions (that can be dismissed in DM) and improves delineation of mass borders, which helps in their characterization. (4) DBT imaging provides location information about lesions without the necessity of additional imaging evaluation in two positions. (5) Compared to other techniques such as MRI, DBT is a relatively low-cos innovation.	(1) The reading time of DBT data could be almost double that of DM. (2) The cost of implementing DBT includes not only the price of the system itself, but also the expense of digital storage capacity to accommodate the large file size of DBT images. (3) Currently, DBT images can be interpreted only on a vendor-specific workstation. (4) The lack of reimbursement for DBT (in some cases). (5) Radiation dose and detection of calcifications are challenging issues which arose in the beginning of DBT.

Other advances are also under investigation: Contrast enhanced DBT is being actively investigated, particularly in terms of imaging technique optimization and quantification of iodine concentration [101-104]; angiotomosynthesis is also currently under development [93]; and combination of DBT with other imaging modalities, such as ultrasounds [105, 106].

SEVERAL STUDIES

Due to the increasing interest in DBT in recent years, there have been many discussions about its true role in breast cancer imaging. Given the advantages already mentioned when compared to 2D mammography, DBT has been referred to as an eventually possibility for replacement of 2D mammography in the breast cancer screening. Its role in diagnostic imaging has also been discussed, mainly for women with dense breasts belonging to high-risk groups.

Table 3 summarizes several studies that have been conducted (2007-2015) identified through a literature review.

These studies presented important results concerning the use and analysis of DBT images. Some studies used 2-view DBT (craniocaudal (CC) and mediolateral oblique (MLO)) while others opted for 1-view DBT. In the latter, the selected 1-view has always been the MLO view because the cancers were considered more obvious in the mammography CC view. Therefore, MLO view for DBT was chosen [32, 107-111]

Image quality was considered as better or equal in 2-view DBT than 2-view conventional mammography and it was inferior mainly in the characterization of microcalcifications [5]. On other study, when a comparison is made between 2-view DM and 2-view DBT, most of the microcalcification clusters were scored similarly [112]. However, a minority was wrong and differently classified in DM and DBT and this fact may have clinical relevance. If a technique is used to allow the viewing of multiple slices together ("slab") using maximum intensity projection within the slab, microcalcifications present a better or equal visibility in most cases (92%) with 1-view DBT than with 2-view DM [109]. In a study comparing breast cancers visibility, cancers were more visible on 1-view DBT than DM (1- and 2-view) [107]. About lesion conspicuity, it was higher for 1-and 2-view DBT when compared to 2-view DM in a general way [32] and in spiculated masses and distortions in particular [113]. Interesting studies on tumor outline and evaluation of lesion size revealed that 1-view DBT was significantly superior than 2-view DM for the lesion determination and evaluation [108, 111].

In all works concerning recall rate with the introduction of DBT, it was shown that DBT+DM decreased the recall rate for non-cancer patients in about 30-40% [5, 114-118]. In fact, this is referred to as one of the added value with the introduction of DBT.

About sensitivity and specificity with the introduction of DBT, it seems that specificity values show some improvements, while sensitivity values are not much changed. Still, the results found are somewhat contradictory: in some studies, the sensitivity values were slightly higher for 2-view DM and specificity values were higher for 2-view DBT [110, 112]; in other studies, there was a higher sensitivity and specificity with 2-view DBT or DBT+DM [114]; and, in other cases, when the values are evaluated specifically for microcalcifications, both sensitivity and specificity values were higher for DM [119].

Regarding clinical performance (measured in some cases as the area under the receiver operating characteristic (ROC) curve), no significant differences were found between 1-view DBT and 2-view DM, 2-view DBT and 2-view DM and 2D synthetized images+DBT and 2-view DBT+ 2-view DM [32, 119-121]. On the other hand, the diagnostic accuracy was proved to be significantly superior with 1-view and 2-view DBT than with 2-view DM [110, 120] and with DBT+DM and DBT+screen-film mammography than with DM and screen-film mammography alone [115, 122].

Besides recall rates, cancer detection rate is another metric referred to as an important potential gain in breast screening with DBT. Despite the fact that, in one singular work, no significant difference in cancer detection rate between DM and DBT+DM was found [117], other studies have shown an increased cancer detection with 2-view DBT [113] or 2-view DBT+2-view DM [116, 118] when compared to DM alone.

The choice of 1-or 2-view DBT and the use of DBT alone or in conjunction with DM are important issues with direct effects in mean interpretation times and average dose levels. Due to its 3D nature, DBT yields more data than DM and more data will need more time to be analyzed. It was shown that DBT examinations with or without DM take about 1.7-3.9 times longer to be interpreted [114, 123, 124]. On the other hand, stand-alone DBT was associated with a much lower to a slightly higher radiation dose compared to that of equivalent DM exams [7, 110]. Therefore, 2-view DBT or DBT+DM exams will be associated with a higher dose than DM alone. Currently, in order to overcome the dose issue, 2D images synthesized from DBT data seems to be a plausible way to acquire only DBT [121, 125]. There are some reasons to acquire both 2D DM and 3D DBT images simultaneously, especially in screening. It is well known that comparison of current images with prior images is standard mammography practice and it is important to detect subtle changes that may be associated with cancer. In addition, the 2D exam is useful for the rapid detection of calcifications and perception of their distribution [95].

SCREENING/CLINICAL TRIALS AND LARGE STUDIES

This section summarizes the main points of the screening/clinical trials and large studies published to date.

Table 3. Summary of studies about DBT in clinical and screening environment

Author/ Ref.	Aim	Equipment	No. Of views	No. Of patients [age range] (mean age)	No. Of readers	Results/Comments
Poplack et al. [5]	Image quality of DBT Vs. CM and estimation of recall rate of screening with DBT+CM	Selenia, Hologic	2-view CM 2-view DBT	98 [34-85] (57 y)	6	• *Image quality* of DBT was equivalent or superior to CM in 89%. It was inferior primarily in the characterization of MCs. • When used adjunctively in screening, DBT would have decreased the *recall rate* by nearly half (~40%).
Andersson et al. [107]	Comparison of breast cancer visibility in 1-view DBT and 1- or 2-view DM	Mammomat, Siemens	1-or 2-view DM 1-view DBT	36 [34-84] (59 y)	2	• If the lesion was equally well seen in both views on DM, the MLO view was chosen for DBT. • The cancers were rated significantly more *visible* on DBT compared to 1-view (22/36) and 2-view (11/36) DM.
Good et al. [123]	Evaluation of diagnostic performance–related issues associated with the interpretation of DBT	Genesis Tomosynthesis System, Hologic	2-view FFDM 2-view DBT	30 n.a.	9	• mode 1: FFDM; mode 2: 11 low-dose projections; mode 3: DBT. • *mean times* (mins) over all examinations: 1.58, 2.03 and 2.72 for mode 1, 2 and 3, respectively. The times were significantly different for the techniques. • The *mean observer performance* values were 0.56, 0.62 and 0.60 for mode 1, 2 and 3, respectively.
Gur et al. [114]	Comparison of diagnostic performance of FFDM with that of DBT	Hologic	2-view FFDM 2-view DBT	125 n.a.	8	• mode 1: FFDM; mode 2: 11 low-dose projections; mode 3: DBT; mode 4: DBT+FFDM. • *Mean times* (mins) to view and rate: 1.22, 1.38, 2.05 and 2.39 for mode 1, 2, 3 and 4 respectively.

Table 3. (Continued)

Author/ Ref.	Aim	Equipment	No. Of views	No. Of patients [age range] (mean age)	No. Of readers	Results/Comments
						• Mode 4: responsible for a significantly reduction of 30% in *recall rate*. Mode 3: responsible for a non-significant reduction of 10% in *recall rate*. • Readers performed at a higher *sensitivity* (n.s.), and *specificity* (sig.) when using mode 3 and mode 4.
Fornvik et al. [108]	Comparison of breast cancer size accuracy with DBT, DM and US	Mammomat Novation, Siemens	2-view DM 1-view DBT (94% MLO)	74 [42-79] (60 y)	1	• *tumor outline* could be determined in significantly more cases with DBT (63) and US (60) than DM (49). • DBT (correlation coef.: 0.86) and US (0.85) *size* correlated well with pathology and significantly better than DM size (0.71). • *Staging* was significantly more accurate with DBT than with DM.
Gennaro et al. [32]	Comparison of clinical performance of DBT and FFDM	GE Healthcare	2-view DM DBT MLO	200 n.a.	6	• *Lesion conspicuity* increases with DBT compared with FFDM. It did not allow a measurable improvement of diagnostic performance. • *Clinical performance* of DBT in 1-view was not inferior to DM in 2-view (same dose).
Kopans et al. [109]	Comparison of MCs clarity on DM and DBT	GE Healthcare	2-view DM DBT MLO	119 n.a.	2	• Slices were grouped together (slab). • *Visibility* of MCs: 41.6% of the cases DBT > DM; 50.4% of the cases DBT = DM; 8% of the cases DBT<DM. • *Clarity* of MCs: 92% of the cases DBT >= DM;
Svane et al. [110]	Comparison of the diagnostic quality,	XC Mammo, XCounter	2-view mammography DBT MLO	144 [40-85] (56.8 y)	2	• The *average dose* used in the DBT was 63% of the 2D-image dose.

Author/ Ref.	Aim	Equipment	No. Of views	No. Of patients [age range] (mean age)	No. Of readers	Results/Comments
	sensitivity, specificity and comfort of 1-view DBT and 2-view					• The *compression force* in DBT was on average about 50% the force used in 2D examination (97% preferred DBT examination). • In 56% of the cases DBT>DM in the *diagnostic quality*. This included the MCs which were rated as having better quality in 41% of the cases. • *sensitivity* was slightly higher for mammography; *specificity* was higher for DBT (n.s. in both).
Spangler et al. [119]	Comparison of detection and characterization of MCs in DBT and FFDM	Selenia, Hologic	2-view FFDM 2-view DBT	100 n.a.	5	• Malignant MCs were *detected* in 90/100 FFDM exams and in 79/99 DBT. • *Specificity* was higher for FFDM (0.71) than for DBT (0.64). Overall MCs detection *sensitivity* was higher for FFDM (0.84) than for DBT (0.75). • *diagnostic performance* as measured by AUC was not significantly different between FFDM and DBT.
Michell et al. [122]	Measurement of diagnostic accuracy of conventional film-screen mammography and FFDM with DBT	Selenia, Hologic	2-view FFDM 2-view DBT	792 n.a.	5	• There was a significant improvement in the *diagnostic accuracy* with the addition of DBT combined with FFDM and film-scree mammography when compared to FFDM plus film-screen mammography and film-screen mammography alone.
Skaane et al. [113]	Comparison of cancer conspicuity and sensitivity of FFDM and DBT	Selenia, Hologic	2-view FFDM 2-view DBT	129 [30-87] (57 y)	3	• FFDM resulted in needle biopsy of 45 breasts: 20 lesions were benign and a total of 25 cancers were diagnosed (84 women were dismissed). • The subsequent DBT interpretation found suspicious findings in 4 of the 84 women dismissed, resulting in 2 cancers (increasing the

Table 3. (Continued)

Author/ Ref.	Aim	Equipment	No. Of views	No. Of patients [age range] (mean age)	No. Of readers	Results/Comments
						cancer detection by 8%). • *conspicuity* were higher for DBT compared to FFDM for cancers presenting as spiculated masses and distortions.
Wallis et al. [120]	Comparison of diagnostic accuracy of FFDM Vs. 2-view and 1-view DBT	MicroDose Mammography, Sectra Mamea	2-view FFDM 1-or 2-view DBT	130 [40-80] (57.3 y)	20	• For *diagnostic accuracy*, FFDM performed significantly worse than 2-view DBT. Significant differences were found for both masses and MCs. • No significant difference in *reader performance* was seen when FFDM was compared with 2-view DBT.
Astley et al. [124]	Comparison of interpretation times in DBT Vs. FFDM	Selenia, Hologic	2-view FFDM 2-view DBT	24-32 cases	4	• The *median time* to interpret FFDM and DBT images was 17.0 secs and 66.0 seconds. The difference was statistically sig. • The readers were relatively inexperienced in DBT interpretation.
Rafferty et al. [115]	Comparison of diagnostic accuracy and recall rates for DBT + DM Vs DM	Selenia, Hologic	2-view DM 2-view DBT	997 [25-80] (51.7 y)	27	• *Diagnostic accuracy* for DBT+DM was superior to that of DM alone. • *Recall rates* for no cancer cases for all readers significantly decreased with addition of DBT.
Mun et al. [111]	Comparison of the accuracy of DBT and FFDM in assessment of	GE Healthcare	2-view FFDM DBT (MLO)	169 [24-76] (50 y)	3	• The percentage of lesions mis-sized at DBT was significantly lower than at FFDM. • There was significantly less mis-sizing at DBT in both heterogeneously and extremely dense breasts.

Author/ Ref.	Aim	Equipment	No. Of views	No. Of patients [age range] (mean age)	No. Of readers	Results/Comments
	local extent of breast cancer.					• DBT was significantly superior to FFDM for the evaluation of *lesion size*.
Zuley et al. [121]	Evaluation of interpretation in 2D syn. images Vs. FFDM images (alone or + DBT)	Selenia, Hologic	2-view DM 2-view DBT	123 [35-74] (51 y)	8	• *Probability of malignancy* (based on the mean AUC) for 2D syn and FFDM images alone was 0.894 and 0.889, respectively (n.s. difference). • *Mean AUC* for 2D syn+DBT and FFDM+DBT was 0.916 and 0.939, respectively (n.s. difference).
McCarthy et al. [116]	Study the impact on screening outcomes for DBT	Selenia, Hologic	2-view DM 2-view DBT	10728 (DM) 15571 (DM+DBT)	6	• DBT screening showed a statistically sig. reduction in *recalls*. • For the entire population, there were sig. fewer recalls with DBT (8.8%) when compared to DM (10.4%) and 0.9/1000 additional *cancers detected*. • In women <50 y. there were sig. fewer recalls with DBT (12.3%) when compared to DM (14%) and 3.6/1000 additional *cancer detected*.
Lourenco et al. [117]	Comparison of recall rate, types of abnormalities recalled, biopsy PPV and cancer detection rate before and after implementation of screening DBT	Selenia, Hologic	n.a.	12577 (DM) 12921 (DM+DBT)	6	• The *recall rate* was 9.3% for DM and 6.4% for DBT (overall sig. reduction of 31%). • The *recall rate* was sig. lower with DM for masses, distortions and MCs. • The *recall rate* was significantly lower with DBT for asymmetries and focal asymmetries. • There was n.s. difference between DM and DBT with regard to *biopsy PPV* or *cancer detection rate*.
Tagliafico et al.	Comparison of DBT and	Selenia, Hologic	2-view DM 2-view DBT	107 (51.7 y)	6	• Estimated *sensitivity* and *specificity* were 100% and 94.6% for FFDM and 91.1% and 100% for

Table 3. (Continued)

Author/ Ref.	Aim	Equipment	No. Of views	No. Of patients [age range] (mean age)	No. Of readers	Results/Comments
[112]	FFDM in the classification of MCs clusters					DBT. • Most MCs clusters were scored similarly on FFDM and DBT. A minority (11/107) of MCs clusters are classified differently on FFDM (benign MC classified as R3) and DBT (malignant MC classified as R2).
Durand et al. [118]	Examination of the recall rates from screening mammography and mammographic findings that caused recall with DBT+DM and DM alone	Selenia, Hologic	2-view DM 2-view DBT	17955 n.a.	7	• The *recall rate* was 7.8% for DM+DBT and 12.3% for DM (36.6% sig. lower in the DM+DBT group). • *Recall rates* for the DM+DBT were sig. lower for patients with asymmetries and MCs. For patients with masses and architectural distortion, the difference in recall rates was n.s. • *Cancer detection* was highest in the DM+DBT group at 5.9/1000 cancers, with 5.7/1000 cancers in the DM group.
Svahn et al. [7]	Comparison of radiation dose levels in DBT and 2- view FFDM	GE Healthc., Siemens, Xcounter, Sectra and Hologic	2-view FFDM 1- or 2-view DBT	n.a.	n.a.	• Stand-alone DBT was associated with a much lower to a slightly higher *radiation dose* compared to that of comparable FFDM units. Dose ratio ranges of 0.34-1.0 for 1-view DBT and 0.68 -1.17 for 2-view DBT. • DBT+ FFDM have dose ratio ranges of 1.03-1.5 for 1-view DBT and 2.0-2.23 for 2-view DBT.

CM: Conventional Mammography, FFDM: Full-field DM, n.s.: not significant, sig.: significant, n.a.: not available, MCs: microcalcifications, AUC: area under the curve, 2D syn.: 2D synthetized, PPV: Positive Predictive Value.

STORM Trial [126]

- Objective: To investigate the effect of integrated DM+DBT in population breast-cancer screening.
- Participants were screened between August 2011 and June 2012.
- Prospective population-based screening trial.
- Dimensions, Hologic system was used.
- Two views (CC and MLO) were obtained of a single breast with DM and DBT.
- 7292 women were included in this study (age range, 48-71 years; median age, 58 years).
- A comparison of mammography screen-reading in two sequential phases (2D DM only versus integrated DM+DBT) was done, yielding paired results for each screening examination.
- 8 radiologists with 3–13 years of experience in screening mammography participated in this study (standard double reading).
- In total, 59 *breast cancers were detected* (including 52 invasive cancers). 0 cancers were detected only by DM, 20 cancers were detected only by DM+DBT and 39 were detected by DM and DM+DBT.
- *Cancer detection rates* were 5.3/1000 and 8.1/1000 for DM and DM+DBT, respectively. It represents a significant increase in cancer detection with DM+DBT.
- In total, there were 395 *false-positive recalls*: 141 occurred with DM, 73 occurred with DM+DBT and 181 with both. The difference found between DM and DM+DBT was significant.
- It is estimated that conditional recall (positive integrated DM+DBT as a condition to recall) could have reduced false-positive recalls by 17.2% without missing any of the cancers detected in the study population.
- Conclusions: Integrated DM+DBT in population breast-cancer screening increases detection of breast cancer and can reduce false-positive recalls.

Haas et al. Study (USA) [127]

- Objective: To compare screening recall rates and cancer detection rates between DM+DBT and DM alone.
- Participants were screened between October 2011 and September 2012.
- Retrospective study conducted in four clinical sites.
- Population-based screening trial.
- Dimensions, Hologic system was used.
- Two views (CC and MLO) were obtained of each breast with DM and DBT.
- 13158 women were included in this study (The mean patient age was 55.8 years for patients screened with DM+DBT and 57.5 years for those screened with DM alone).
- 8 radiologists with 2–23 years of experience in screening mammography participated in this study.
- The *overall recall rates* were 12% and 8.4% for DM and DM+DBT, respectively. It represents a 30% significative decrease in overall recall rates for DM+DBT.
- DM+DBT reduced *recall rates* for all breast density and patient age groups, with significance differences for: scattered fibroglandular breasts, heterogeneously and extremely dense breasts, patients younger than 40 years, those aged 40–49 years, those aged 50–59 years, and those aged 60–69 years.
- *Cancer detection rates* were 5.2/1000 and 5.7/1000 for DM and DM+DBT, respectively. In doesn't represent a significative increase in cancer detection rates for DM+DBT.
- Conclusions: Patients undergoing DM+DBT had significantly lower screening recall rates. The greatest reductions were for those younger than 50 years and those with dense breasts. A nonsignificant increase in cancer detection was observed in the DM+DBT group.

Rose et al. Study (USA) [128]

- Objective: To assess the changes in performance measures after the introduction of DBT systems into clinical practice.

- The analysis compares the outcomes of screening mammography studies interpreted in 2010 before the introduction of DBT to results acquired after the introduction of DBT during the period of May 2011 to the end of January 2012.

- It is an observational single-site study which uses verified practice- and outcome-related databases.

- Dimensions, Hologic system was used.

- Two views (CC and MLO) were obtained of each breast with DM and DBT.

- The radiation doses used for DM and DBT are approximately the same. Thus, the radiation dose when DM+DBT images were obtained was approximately twice that used for DM.

- 23355 women were included in this study. 13856 screening examinations with DM (mean age, 53.8 years) and 9499 screening examinations with DM+DBT (mean age, 54.5 years).

- 6 radiologists with 2–32 years of experience in screening mammography participated in this study.

- *Recall rates* were 8.7% and 5.5% for DM and DM+DBT, respectively. It represents a significative decrease recall rates for DM+DBT.

- *Recall rates* decreased for all breast density categories and age groups.

- *Biopsy rates* (biopsies that resulted from a recalled case) were 15.2/1000 and 13.5/1000 for DM and DM+DBT, respectively. It doesn't represent a significative decrease in biopsy rates for DM+DBT.

- *Cancer detection rates* were 4.0/1000 and 5.4/1000 for DM and DM+DBT, respectively. It doesn't represent a significative increase in cancer detection rates for DM+DBT. The *invasive cancer detection rates* were 2.8/1000 and 4.3/1000 for DM and DM+DBT, respectively. It doesn't represent a significative increase in invasive cancer detection rates for DM + DBT.

- The *positive predictive values for recalls* were 4.7% and 10.1% for DM and DM+DBT, respectively. It represents a significative increase in positive predictive values for recalls for DM+DBT.

- The *positive predictive values for biopsies* were 26.5% and 39.8% for DM and DM+DBT, respectively. It doesn't represent a significative increase in positive predictive values for biopsied for DM + DBT.

- Conclusions: implementation of DBT in screening practice resulted in a consistent significant improvement in performance. The positive predictive values of recalls doubled with the addition of DBT. Improved performance resulted in significant decreases in recall rates and simultaneous increases in cancer detection rates, in particular those of invasive cancers.

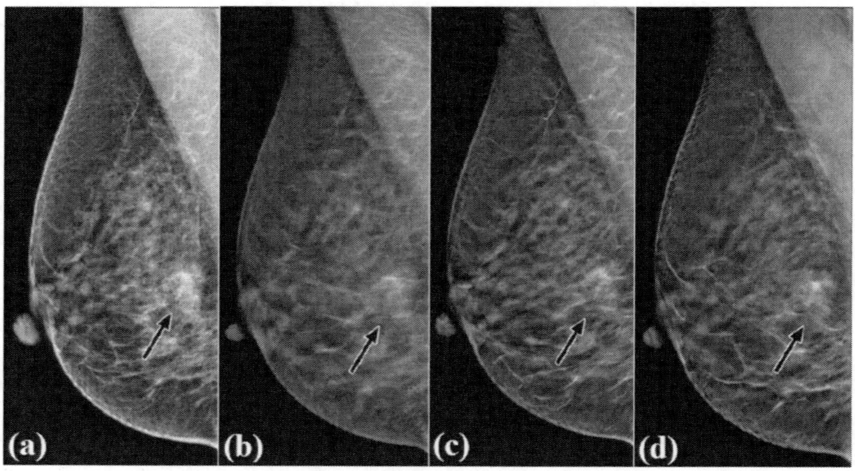

Figure 7. DM image (**a**) demonstrate a suspicious area. Three DBT slice images (b-d) show that structures at different levels in breast can summate to create suspicious region on DM image that may be identified as negative or superimposed tissue on DBT images [128].

Oslo Trial [129-131]

- Study start date: November 2010; Estimated study completion date: September 2015.
- The study was divided into two periods: period 1 from November 2010 to December 2011 and period 2 from January 2012 to December 2012.
- First large scale trial to implement DBT.
- Single institution prospective, reader- and modality-balanced screening study.
- Population-based screening trial.
- Dimensions, Hologic system was used.

- Two views (CC and MLO) were obtained of each breast with DM and DBT.
- The radiation dose levels for DM+DBT were approximately twice those for DM alone.
- 24901 women were included in this study (age range, 50-69 years; mean age, 59.2 years). Study population of period 1: 12631 women; study population of period 2: 12270 women.

- Four arms study: (1) conventional DM; (2) DM + CAD; (3) DM + DBT; and (4) synthetic 2D + DBT.
- 8 radiologists with 2–31 years of experience in screening mammography participated in this study. Images were interpreted independently by 4 radiologists by using each of the reading modes.
- Consensus-based arbitration meeting: All cases received at least one score of 2 ("recalled for a probably benign finding") or greater in at least one arm were discussed at arbitration before a consensus-based clinical treatment decision was made.

Study 1 [130]

- Objective: To assess cancer detection rates, false-positive rates before arbitration, positive predictive values for women recalled after arbitration, and the type of cancers detected with use of DM alone and combined with DBT.
- Arm 1 Vs. arm 3: conventional DM Vs. DM+DBT.
- Study carried out during period 1.
- *Cancer detection rates* were 6.1/1000 and 8.0/1000 for DM and DM+DBT, respectively. It represents a 27% significative increase in cancer detection rates for DM+DBT. 25 additional *invasive cancers* (40% significative increase) were detected with DM+DBT.
- Before arbitration, *false-positive rates* were 61.1/1000 and 53.1/1000 for DM and DM+DBT, respectively. It represents a 15% significative decrease in false-positive rates for DM+DBT.
- After arbitration, *positive predictive values* for recalled patients with cancer proven later were 29.1% and 28.5% for DM and DM+DBT, respectively (it doesn't represent a significative decrease for DM+DBT).

- The *mean interpretation times* were 45 seconds and 91 seconds for DM and DM+DBT, respectively. It represents a significative increase for DM+DBT.
- Conclusions: There was a significant increase in cancer detection rates, particularly for invasive cancers and a simultaneous decrease in false-positive rates with DM+DBT compared to DM alone.

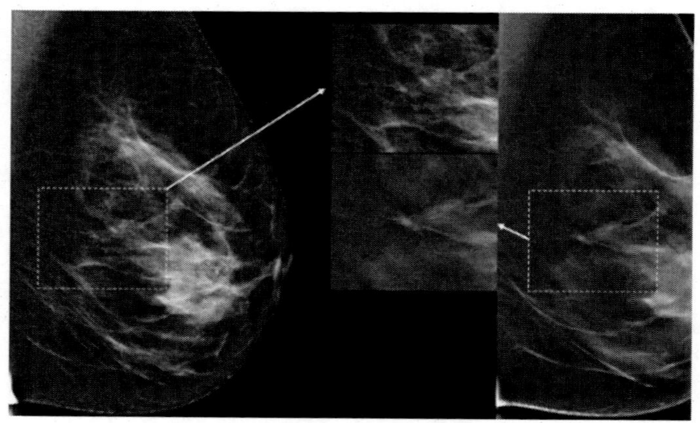

Figure 8. MLO views of left breast. Left: Mammogram shows normal findings (score 1); Right: DBT image demonstrates spiculated mass (score 3). An 8-mm invasive ductal carcinoma was diagnosed at histologic examination [130].

Study 2 [129]

- Objective: To compare double readings when interpreting DM and DBT during mammographic screening.
- Paired double reading of 2D (conventional DM and DM+CAD) and 2D+3D (DM+DBT and synthetic 2D+DBT) were analyzed.
- Study carried out during period 1.
- Before arbitration, the *false-positive rates* were 10.3% and 8.5% for 2D and 2D+3D, respectively. It represents a 18% significative decrease in false-positive rates for 2D+3D.
- *Recall rates* were 2.9% and 3.7% for 2D and 2D+3D, respectively. It represents a significative increase in recall rates for 2D+3D. The 2D+3D approach resulted in the detection of 29 additional cancers.
- *Cancer detection rates* were 7.1/1000 and 9.4/1000 for 2D and 2D+3D, respectively. It represents a 30% significative increase in cancer detection rates with 2D+3D.

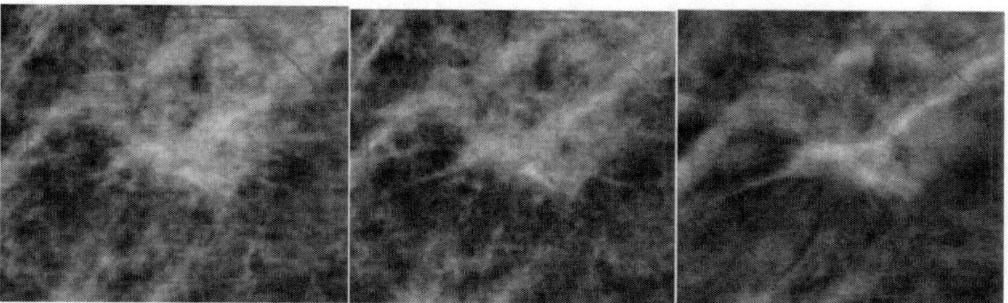

Figure 9. A CC view. Enlargement of the 2D (left) and synthesized 2D (middle) shows a suspicious but no conclusive irregular density. On DBT image enlargement (right), a spiculated mass consistent with invasive cancer is clearly seen. Histology revealed an 8-mm invasive lobular carcinoma grade 2 [129].

- The *positive predictive values* for the verified attributable cancers per recalls were 24.7% and 25.5% for 2D and 2D+3D, respectively (it doesn't represent a significative increase for 2D+3D).
- The *mean interpretation times* were 48 seconds and 89 seconds for 2D and 2D+3D, respectively. It represents a significative increase for 2D+3D.
- The *average mean fibroglandular doses* were 1.58 mGy, 1.95 mGy and 3.52 mGy for DM, synthetic 2D + DBT and DM + DBT.
- Conclusions: The double reading using DBT-based imaging (DM + DBT and synthetic 2D+DBT) resulted in a significant increase in cancer detection rates (especially in the detection of invasive, node-negative cancers) and simultaneously a reduction in false-positive rates compared with the double reading of 2D imaging alone (DM and DM + CAD).

Study 3 [131]

- Objective: To compare the performance of two versions of reconstructed 2D images (synthetic 2D) in combination with DBT versus the performance of standard DM + DBT.
- Study carried out during period 1 and 2.
- The synthetic 2D images used in the first period were reconstructed by using an early version of the image reconstruction software. An improved version that uses section-weighted summation and enhanced features was installed after and this version was used for examinations performed during period 2.

- DM + DBT Vs. synthetic 2D+DBT in period 1 and period 2.
- *False-positive rates* were 5.3% and 4.6% for DM+DBT and synthetic 2D + DBT, respectively, for period 1. It represents a significant decrease for synthetic 2D+DBT in period 1.
- *False-positive rates* were 4.6% and 4.5% for DM+DBT and synthetic 2D + DBT, respectively, for period 2. it doesn't represent a significative decrease for synthetic 2D+DBT in period 2.
- *Cancer detection rates* were 8/1000 and 7.4/1000 for DM+DBT and synthetic 2D + DBT, respectively, for period 1. it doesn't represent a significative decrease for synthetic 2D+DBT in period 1.
- *Cancer detection rates* were 7.8/1000 and 7.7/1000 for DM+DBT and synthetic 2D+DBT, respectively, for period 2. it doesn't represent a significative decrease for synthetic 2D+DBT in period 2.
- The *positive predictive values* of verified attributable cancers per number of recalls were 28.5% and 30.3% for DM+DBT and synthetic 2D+DBT, respectively, for period 1. it doesn't represent a significative increase for synthetic 2D+DBT in period 1.
- The *positive predictive values* of verified attributable cancers per number of recalls were 32.1% and 34.9% for DM+DBT and synthetic 2D+DBT, respectively, for period 2. it doesn't represent a significative increase for synthetic 2D+DBT in period 2.
- During period 1, synthetic 2D+DBT showed relatively high performance levels, although not as high as the performance achieved by DM+DBT. During period 2, the performance of synthetic 2D+DBT images was reasonably comparable to that of DM+DBT.
- Conclusions: synthetic 2D+DBT performed comparably to DM+DBT when interpreting screening mammograms in terms of cancer detection rates and false-positive rates.

Friedewald et al. Study (USA) [132]

- Objective: To determine if mammography combined with tomosynthesis is associated with better performance of breast screening programs in the United States.
- This study compared performance of breast cancer screening before and after introduction of DBT over 2 periods.: period 1 where DM screening examinations were done 1 year before DBT implementation (from March 2010 - October 2011until the date of DBT

implementation); period 2 where DM+DBT examinations were done (from March 2011 - October 2012 until December 2012).

- Retrospective study conducted in 13 centers.
- The study with the largest number of centers and participants.
- Dimensions, Hologic system was used.
- Two views (CC and MLO) were obtained of each breast with DM and DBT.

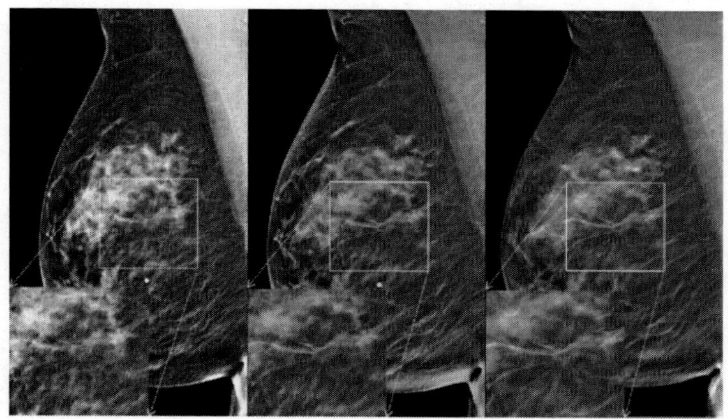

Figure 10. Left: DM image. Middle: synthesized 2D image (period 2). Right: DBT image. Reader scores for the study were 1 for DM, 3 for DM+DBT, and 4 for synthetic 2D+DBT [131].

- 454850 women were included in this study. The mean age of patients undergoing imaging with DM alone was 57.0 years (range, 54.4-60.5 years) and with DM+DBT was 56.2 years (range, 52.6-59.7 years).
- 139 radiologists with experience in screening mammography participated in this study.
- *Recall rates* were 107/1000 and 91/1000 for DM and DM+DBT, respectively. It represents a significative decrease in recall rates for DM+DBT.
- *Biopsies rates* were 18.1/1000 and 19.3/1000 for DM and DM+DBT, respectively. It represents a significative increase in biopsies rates for DM+DBT.
- *Cancer detection rates* were 4.2/1000 and 5.4/1000 for DM and DM+DBT, respectively. It represents a significative increase in cancer detection rates for DM+DBT. For *invasive cancer detection rates*, values of 2.9/1000 and 4.1/1000 were found for DM+DBT,

respectively. It represents a significative increase in invasive cancer detection rates for DM+DBT. The rate of in *situ cancer detection* was 1.4/1000 for both modalities.

- The mean *positive predictive values for recall* were 4.3% and 6.4% for DM and DM+DBT, respectively. It represents a significative increase in positive predictive values for recall for DM+DBT.
- The mean *positive predictive values for biopsies* were 24.2% and 29.2% for DM and DM+DBT, respectively. It represents a significative increase in positive predictive values for biopsies for DM+DBT.
- Conclusions: The addition of DBT to DM was associated with a significative decrease in recall rate and an increase in cancer detection rate.

Malmo Trial [133]

- Objective: To assess the performance of 1-view DBT in breast cancer screening.
- Study start date: March 2010; Estimated study completion date: December 2017.
- Until now, the known results are from an explorative analysis of the first half of the study population.
- Single institution prospective screening study.
- Population-based screening trial.
- Mammomat Inspiration, Siemens system was used.
- 7500 women were included in this study (age range, 40-74 years; mean age, 56 years). The whole study should to account for 15000 participants.
- In practice it studies three approaches: (1) 1-view DBT Vs. 2-view DM; (2) 1-view DBT Vs. 1-view DM and (3) 2-view DM alone.
- 6 radiologists with 8–41 years of experience in breast imaging participated in this study. The reading included blinded double reading and scoring in two independent reading arms: DBT arm (1 and 2 of previous point) and DM arm (3 of previous point).
- If one or both of the screening modalities was given a score of 3 or higher by one of the two readers, it was referred for arbitration, where at least two readers re-evaluated the images and decided whether to

recall the woman for further work-up, irrespective of the score on the other modality.

- The DBT examinations were performed with *reduced compression* of the breast compared to the acquired DM image set, with a goal of a 50% reduction. This was achieved in most cases (about 90%), but sometimes more pressure was needed to keep especially large breasts in a proper position for the MLO projection.

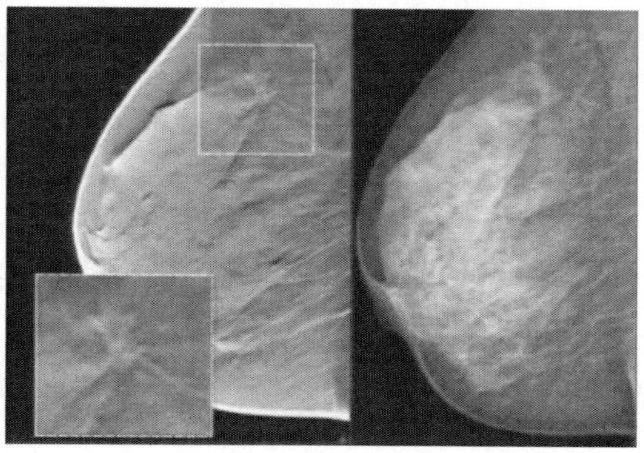

Figure 11. Left: DBT image; right: DM image. Cancer detected by DBT alone (left). A 15-mm invasive ductal carcinoma, histological grade 1 and lymph node negative, was diagnosed at histological examination [133].

- *Breast cancer was detected* in 68 women: 1 cancer was detected only by DM arm, 21 cancers were detected only by DBT arm (including 17 invasive cancers) and 46 were detected by both arms. Cancers detected by DBT arm alone were found in both dense and fatty breasts.
- *Cancer detection rates* were 6.3/1000 and 8.9/1000 for DM arm and DBT arm, respectively. It represents a 43% significative increase in cancer detection rates for DBT arm.
- After arbitration, *recall rates* were 2.6% and 3.8% for DM arm and DBT arm, respectively. It represents a 43% significative increase in cancer detection rates for DBT arm. The increase in recall rate for DBT arm is justified by the fact that DBT enhances benign lesions and sometimes islands of normal breast parenchyma.
- The *positive predictive values* were 24% for both arms.
- The *radiation dose* for 1-view DBT examination was lower than an ordinary 2-view DM screen.
- The reduced *compression force* was much appreciated by the women.

- Conclusions: There was a significant increase in cancer detection rate and recall rate when 1-view DBT as a stand-alone screening modality compared to 2-view DM.

TOMMY Trial [134]

- Objective: (1) To compare the diagnostic accuracy of using DM+DBT or synthetic 2D+DBT Vs. standard 2D DM alone; (2) To determine if the use of DM+DBT or synthetic 2D+DBT improves the accuracy of detection of: small or subtle breast cancers, cancers in women with dense breasts, cancers presenting as soft-tissue masses and cancers presenting as microcalcifications; (3) To assess the performance of two automated breast density software programs against observer-based visually assessed breast density; (4) To assess the association of breast density with cancer incidence.
- Participants were recruited between July 2011 and March 20123.
- Retrospective reading study conducted in six United Kingdom centers.
- Women (aged 47–73 years) recalled for further assessment after routine breast screening and women (aged 40–49 years) with moderate/high of risk of developing breast cancer who were attending annual mammography screening were recruited into the trial.
- Dimensions, Hologic system was used.
- Two views (CC and MLO) were obtained of each breast with DM and DBT.
- 8869 women were included in this study.
- The number of readers available varied from week to week; the average number per week was 16, with variable years of experience.
- Readers reviewed (1) DM, (2) DM+DBT or (3) synthetic 2D+DBT images for a case without access to original screening mammograms or prior examinations, and readers were blinded to the outcome status of each case.
- *Overall sensitivity* was 87%, 89% and 88% for DM, DM+DBT and synthetic 2D+DBT, respectively. The difference in sensitivity between DM and DM+DBT was of borderline and for synthetic 2D+DBT there was no significant difference.
- *Sensitivity for invasive tumor of size 11-20 mm* was 86%, 93% and 91% for DM, DM+DBT and synthetic 2D+DBT, respectively. It was

significantly higher for DM+DBT and synthetic 2D+DBT than for DM.

- *Sensitivity for breast density of 50% or more* was 86%, 93% and 87% for DM, DM+DBT and synthetic 2D+DBT, respectively. It was significantly higher for DM+DBT than for DM.
- *Sensitivity for grade 2 invasive tumors* was 87%, 91% and 88% for DM, DM+DBT and synthetic 2D+DBT, respectively. It was significantly higher for DM+DBT than for DM.
- *Sensitivity where the dominant radiological feature was a mass* was 89%, 92% and 91% for DM, DM+DBT and synthetic 2D+DBT, respectively. It was significantly higher for DM+DBT than for DM.
- *Overall specificity* was 58%, 69% and 71% for DM, DM+DBT and synthetic 2D+DBT, respectively. It was significantly higher for DM+DBT and for synthetic 2D+DBT than for DM.
- The increased *specificity* with DM+DBT and synthetic 2D+DBT was observed in all subgroups of density and dominant radiological feature and across all age groups. In all three modalities, specificity tended to be lower for microcalcifications and higher for distortion and asymmetry. Still, the significant improvement in specificity for both DM+DBT and synthetic 2D+DBT was consistently observed in these categories.
- With ROC analysis, a significant increase in *diagnostic accuracy* for DM+DBT and synthetic 2D+DBT compared with DM alone was observed (most likely as a result of the marked improvement in specificity).
- Conclusions: Specificity of DM+DBT and synthetic 2D+DBT was better than DM alone but there was only marginal improvement in sensitivity. The performance of synthetic 2D+DBT appeared to be compared to standard DM.

Reader Study

- Objective: to establish whether or not increased experience of reading DBT images altered performance in terms of recall rate and cancer detection.
- Conclusions: The lack of change over time indicates that a larger set of training images is probably unnecessary, although the intersite variations indicate that individuals operate according to local practice even under test conditions.

Breast Density Assessment Study

- Objective: to evaluate and utilize two of the commercially available software packages for the measurement of volumetric breast density and compare these with observer-based scores of area density. This data is used to determine if the addition of DBT improved the detection of cancers in women at higher risk of developing breast cancer due to increased breast density. A secondary aim of this study was to assess whether or not there is a relationship between breast density and breast cancer incidence.
- Conclusions: Analysis of the relationship between cancer incidence and volumetric density has shown that there is a significant association of increased risk with density. A lack of correlation between observer scores of breast density and automated analysis was observed.

CONCLUSION

In general, studies demonstrated the DBT's potential to reduce recall rates and increase cancer detection rates. Based on the same methodology, it would be interesting to make a comparison between the different DBT systems present in the market or approved by FDA.

The impact on interval cancers and mortality from breast cancer from screening with DBT has not yet been reported. However, the added value from DBT in early detection of breast cancer is marked, being one useful tool from breast cancer screening.

ACKNOWLEDGMENTS

This work was supported in part by Fundação para a Ciência e a Tecnologia - Portugal (projects Pest-OE/SAU/IU0645/2013, Pest-OE/SAU/IU0645/2014 and PTDC/BBB-IMG/3310/2012).

REFERENCES

[1] Sudhakar, A. History of Cancer, Ancient and Modern Treatment Methods. *Journal of cancer science & therapy*, 2009, **1**(2), pp. 1-4.

[2] *Cancer Fact sheet N°297.* [cited 2016 March]; Available from: http://www.who.int/mediacentre/factsheets/fs297/en/.

[3] Siegel, RL; Miller, KD; Jemal, A. Cancer statistics, 2016. *CA Cancer J Clin*, 2016, 66(1), pp. 7-30.

[4] Berry, DA; et al., Effect of screening and adjuvant therapy on mortality from breast cancer. *N Engl J Med*, 2005, 353(17), pp. 1784-92.

[5] Poplack, SP; et al., Digital breast tomosynthesis: initial experience in 98 women with abnormal digital screening mammography. *AJR Am J Roentgenol*, 2007, 189(3), pp. 616-23.

[6] Hubbard, RA; et al., Cumulative probability of false-positive recall or biopsy recommendation after 10 years of screening mammography: a cohort study. *Ann Intern Med*, 2011, 155(8), pp. 481-92.

[7] Svahn, TM; et al., Review of radiation dose estimates in digital breast tomosynthesis relative to those in two-view full-field digital mammography. *Breast*, 2015, 24(2), pp. 93-99.

[8] Sechopoulos, I. A review of breast tomosynthesis. Part I. The image acquisition process. *Med Phys*, 2013, 40(1), pp. 014301.

[9] Brandt, KR; et al., Can digital breast tomosynthesis replace conventional diagnostic mammography views for screening recalls without calcifications? A comparison study in a simulated clinical setting. *AJR Am J Roentgenol*, 2013, 200(2), pp. 291-8.

[10] Kopans, DB. Digital breast tomosynthesis from concept to clinical care. *AJR Am J Roentgenol*, 2014, 202(2), pp. 299-308.

[11] *Early history of cancer.* [cited 2016 March]; Available from: http://www.cancer.org/cancer/cancerbasics/thehistoryofcancer/the-history-of-cancer-what-is-cancer.

[12] *10 Must-Know 2015 Global Cancer Facts.* [cited 2016 March]; Available from: http://www.cancer.org/research/acsresearchupdates/more/10-must-know-2015-global-cancer-facts.

[13] Holford, TR; et al., Changing patterns in breast cancer incidence trends. *J Natl Cancer Inst Monogr*, 2006(36), pp. 19-25.

[14] *Breast cancer survival rates, by stage.* [cited 2016 March]; Available from: http://www.cancer.org/cancer/breastcancer/detailedguide/breast-cancer-survival-by-stage.

[15] Nover, AB; et al., Modern Breast Cancer Detection: A Technological Review. *International Journal of Biomedical Imaging*, 2009, 2009.

[16] Kosters, JP; Gotzsche, PC. Regular self-examination or clinical examination for early detection of breast cancer. *Cochrane Database Syst Rev*, 2003(2), pp. Cd003373.

[17] Bassett, LW; Gold, RH. The evolution of mammography. *American Journal of Roentgenology*, 1988, 150(3), pp. 493-498.

[18] Karellas, A; Vedantham, S. Breast cancer imaging: a perspective for the next decade. *Med Phys*, 2008, 35(11), pp. 4878-97.

[19] Shapiro, S; Strax, P; Venet, L. Periodic breast cancer screening in reducing mortality from breast cancer. *Jama*, 1971, 215(11), pp. 1777-85.

[20] Thurfjell, EL; Lindgren, JA. Breast cancer survival rates with mammographic screening: similar favorable survival rates for women younger and those older than 50 years. *Radiology*, 1996, 201(2), pp. 421-6.

[21] Hendrick, RE; et al., Benefit of screening mammography in women aged 40-49: a new meta-analysis of randomized controlled trials. *J Natl Cancer Inst Monogr*, 1997(22), pp. 87-92.

[22] Tabar, L; et al., Beyond randomized controlled trials: organized mammographic screening substantially reduces breast carcinoma mortality. *Cancer*, 2001, 91(9), pp. 1724-31.

[23] Reduction in breast cancer mortality from organized service screening with mammography: 1. Further confirmation with extended data. *Cancer Epidemiol Biomarkers Prev*, 2006, 15(1), pp. 45-51.

[24] Reduction in breast cancer mortality from the organised service screening with mammography: 2. Validation with alternative analytic methods. *Cancer Epidemiol Biomarkers Prev*, 2006, 15(1),pp.52-6.

[25] Lewin, JM; et al., Comparison of full-field digital mammography with screen-film mammography for cancer detection: results of 4,945 paired examinations. *Radiology*, 2001, 218(3), pp. 873-80.

[26] Pisano, ED; et al., Diagnostic performance of digital versus film mammography for breast-cancer screening. *N Engl J Med*, 2005. 353(17), pp. 1773-83.

[27] Skaane, P; Hofvind, S; Skjennald, A. Randomized trial of screen-film versus full-field digital mammography with soft-copy reading in population-based screening program: follow-up and final results of Oslo II study. *Radiology*, 2007, 244(3), pp. 708-17.

[28] Pisano, ED; et al., Diagnostic accuracy of digital versus film mammography: exploratory analysis of selected population subgroups in DMIST. *Radiology*, 2008, 246(2), pp. 376-83.

[29] *FDA - Digital Accreditation*. [cited 2016 March]; Available from: http://www.fda.gov/Radiation-EmittingProducts/MammographyQuality StandardsActandProgram/FacilityCertificationandInspection/ucm114148 .htm.

[30] Bick, U; Diekmann, F. *Digital Mammography*. 2010: Springer Berlin Heidelberg.

[31] Lindfors, KK; et al., Dedicated breast CT: initial clinical experience. *Radiology*, 2008, 246(3), pp. 725-33.

[32] Gennaro, G; et al., Digital breast tomosynthesis versus digital mammography: a clinical performance study. *Eur Radiol*, 2010, 20(7), pp. 1545-53.

[33] Stavros, AT; Rapp, CL; Parker, SH. *Breast Ultrasound.*, 2004, Lippincott Williams & Wilkins.

[34] Berg, WA; et al., Combined screening with ultrasound and mammography vs mammography alone in women at elevated risk of breast cancer. *Jama*, 2008, 299(18), pp. 2151-63.

[35] Kelly, KM; et al., Breast cancer detection using automated whole breast ultrasound and mammography in radiographically dense breasts. *Eur Radiol*, 2010, 20(3), pp. 734-42.

[36] Corsetti, V; et al., Evidence of the effect of adjunct ultrasound screening in women with mammography-negative dense breasts: interval breast cancers at 1 year follow-up. *Eur J Cancer*, 2011, 47(7), pp. 1021-6.

[37] Teh, W; Wilson, AR. The role of ultrasound in breast cancer screening. A consensus statement by the European Group for Breast Cancer Screening. *Eur J Cancer*, 1998, 34(4), pp. 449-50.

[38] Chiou, SY; et al., Sonographic features of nonpalpable breast cancer: a study based on ultrasound-guided wire-localized surgical biopsies. *Ultrasound Med Biol*, 2006, 32(9), pp. 1299-306.

[39] Zhi, H; et al., Comparison of ultrasound elastography, mammography, and sonography in the diagnosis of solid breast lesions. *J Ultrasound Med*, 2007, 26(6), pp. 807-15.

[40] Sehgal, CM; et al., A review of breast ultrasound. *J Mammary Gland Biol Neoplasia*, 2006, 11(2), pp. 113-23.

[41] Stelling, CB; et al., Prototype coil for magnetic resonance imaging of the female breast. Work in progress. *Radiology*, 1985, 154(2), pp. 457-62.

[42] Kuhl, C. The Current Status of Breast MR Imaging Part I. Choice of Technique, Image Interpretation, Diagnostic Accuracy, and Transfer to Clinical Practice. *Radiology*, 2007, 244(2), pp. 356-378.

[43] Orel, SG; Schnall, MD. MR Imaging of the Breast for the Detection, Diagnosis, and Staging of Breast Cancer. *Radiology*, 2001, 220(1), pp. 13-30.

[44] Planche, K; Vinnicombe, S. Breast imaging in the new era. *Cancer Imaging*, 2004, 4(2), pp. 39-50.

[45] Mann, RM; et al., Breast MRI: guidelines from the European Society of Breast Imaging. *European Radiology*, 2008, 18(7), pp. 1307-1318.

[46] Sardanelli, F; et al., Sensitivity of MRI Versus Mammography for Detecting Foci of Multifocal, Multicentric Breast Cancer in Fatty and Dense Breasts Using the Whole-Breast Pathologic Examination as a Gold Standard. *American Journal of Roentgenology*, 2004, 183(4), pp. 1149-1157.

[47] Leach, MO. Application of magnetic resonance imaging to angiogenesis in breast cancer. *Breast Cancer Res*, 2001, 3(1), pp. 22-7.

[48] Kuhl, CK. Current Status of Breast MR Imaging Part 2. Clinical Applications. *Radiology*, 2007, 244(3), pp. 672-691.

[49] Saslow, D; et al., American Cancer Society guidelines for breast screening with MRI as an adjunct to mammography. *CA Cancer J Clin*, 2007, 57(2), pp. 75-89.

[50] Sree, SV; et al., Breast imaging: A survey. *World Journal of Clinical Oncology*, 2011, 2(4), pp. 171-178.

[51] Moore, SG. et al., Cost-effectiveness of MRI compared to mammography for breast cancer screening in a high risk population. *BMC Health Serv Res*, 2009, 9, p. 9.

[52] Avril, N; et al., Breast imaging with positron emission tomography and fluorine-18 fluorodeoxyglucose: use and limitations. *J Clin Oncol*, 2000, 18(20), pp. 3495-502.

[53] Thompson, CJ; et al., Feasibility study for positron emission mammography. *Med Phys*, 1994, 21(4), pp. 529-38.

[54] Doshi, NK; et al., Design and evaluation of an LSO PET detector for breast cancer imaging. *Medical Physics*, 2000, 27(7), pp.1535-1543.

[55] Raylman, RR; et al. An apparatus for positron emission mammography-guided breast biopsy. in Engineering in Medicine and Biology Society, 2000. *Proceedings of the 22nd Annual International Conference of the IEEE.*, 2000.

[56] Turkington, TG; et al. A large field of view positron emission mammography imager. in *Nuclear Science Symposium Conference Record, 2002 IEEE.*, 2002.

[57] Wollenweber, SD; et al. Investigation of the quantitative capabilities of a positron emission mammography system. in *Nuclear Science Symposium Conference Record, 2004 IEEE.*, 2004.

[58] Wang, GC; et al., Characterization of the LBNL PEM camera. *IEEE Transactions on Nuclear Science*, 2006, 53(3), pp. 1129-1135.

[59] Amaral, P; et al., Performance and quality control of Clear-PEM detector modules. *Nuclear Instruments and Methods in Physics Research Section A: Accelerators, Spectrometers, Detectors and Associated Equipment*, 2007, 580(2), pp. 1123-1126.

[60] Fowler, AM. A molecular approach to breast imaging. *J Nucl Med*, 2014, 55(2), pp. 177-80.

[61] Glass, SB; Shah, ZA. Clinical utility of positron emission mammography. *Proceedings (Baylor University. Medical Center)*, 2013, 26(3), pp. 314-319.

[62] Berg, WA; et al., Comparative effectiveness of positron emission mammography and MRI in the contralateral breast of women with newly diagnosed breast cancer. *AJR Am J Roentgenol*, 2012, 198(1), pp. 219-32.

[63] Boone, JM; et al., Computed tomography for imaging the breast. *J Mammary Gland Biol Neoplasia*, 2006, 11(2), pp. 103-11.

[64] Prionas, ND; et al., Contrast-enhanced dedicated breast CT: initial clinical experience. *Radiology*, 2010, 256(3), pp. 714-23.

[65] Lindfors, KK; et al., Dedicated breast CT: The optimal cross sectional imaging solution? *Radiologic clinics of North America*, 2010, 48(5), pp. 1043-1054.

[66] McKinley, RL; et al. Investigation of cone-beam acquisitions implemented using a novel dedicated mammotomography system with unique arbitrary orbit capability (Honorable Mention Poster Award)., 2005.

[67] Ning, R; et al. *A novel cone beam breast CT scanner: system evaluation.*, 2007.

[68] Dobbins, JT. 3rd, Tomosynthesis imaging: at a translational crossroads. *Med Phys*, 2009, 36(6), pp. 1956-67.

[69] Reiser, I; Glick, S. *Tomosynthesis Imaging.*, 2014, Taylor & Francis.

[70] Ziedses des Plantes, BG. Seriescopy, Een Rontgenographische method welke het mogelijk maakt achtereenvolgens een oneindig aantal

evenwijdige vlakken van het te onderzoeken voorwerp afzonderlijk te beschouwen (Seriescopy, a Roentgenographic method which allows an infinite number of successive parallel planes of the test object to be considered separately) (English Translation). *Ned. Tijdschr*, 1935, Geneesk 51, 5852–5856.

[71] Grant, DG. Tomosynthesis: A Three-Dimensional Radiographic Imaging Technique. *IEEE Transactions on Biomedical Engineering*, 1972, BME-19(1), pp. 20-28.

[72] Webber, RL; et al., Comparison of film, direct digital, and tuned-aperture computed tomography images to identify the location of crestal defects around endosseous titanium implants. *Oral Surg Oral Med Oral Pathol Oral Radiol Endod*, 1996, 81(4), pp. 480-90.

[73] Niklason, LT; et al., Digital tomosynthesis in breast imaging. *Radiology*, 1997, 205(2), pp. 399-406.

[74] Dobbins, JTI; Webber, RL; Hames, SM. Tomosynthesis for improved pulmonary nodule detection (abstract). *Radiology*, 1998, 209(P):280.

[75] Wu, T; et al., Tomographic mammography using a limited number of low-dose cone-beam projection images. *Med Phys*, 2003, 30(3), pp. 365-80.

[76] Godfrey, DJ; McAdams, HP; Dobbins, JT. 3rd, Optimization of the matrix inversion tomosynthesis (MITS) impulse response and modulation transfer function characteristics for chest imaging. *Med Phys*, 2006, 33(3), pp. 655-67.

[77] Zhou, J; Zhao, B; Zhao, W. A computer simulation platform for the optimization of a breast tomosynthesis system. *Med Phys*, 2007, 34(3), pp. 1098-109.

[78] Deller, T; et al. Effect of acquisition parameters on image quality in digital tomosynthesis., 2007.

[79] Zhao, W; et al. Optimization of detector operation and imaging geometry for breast tomosynthesis., 2007.

[80] Gifford, HC; et al. *Optimizing breast-tomosynthesis acquisition parameters with scanning model observers.*, 2008.

[81] Reiser, I; Lau, BA; Nishikawa, RM. Effect of Scan Angle and Reconstruction Algorithm on Model Observer Performance in Tomosynthesis, in Digital Mammography: 9th International Workshop, IWDM 2008 Tucson, AZ, USA, July 20-23, 2008 Proceedings, E.A. Krupinski, Editor. 2008, Springer Berlin Heidelberg: Berlin, Heidelberg. pp. 606-611.

[82] Chan, HP; et al., Detection of Masses in Digital Breast Tomosynthesis Mammography: Effects of the Number of Projection Views and Dose, in Digital Mammography: 9th International Workshop, IWDM 2008 Tucson, AZ, USA, July 20-23, 2008 Proceedings, E.A. Krupinski, Editor. 2008, Springer Berlin Heidelberg: Berlin, Heidelberg. pp. 279-285.

[83] Sechopoulos, I; Ghetti, C. Optimization of the acquisition geometry in digital tomosynthesis of the breast. *Med Phys*, 2009, 36(4), pp. 1199-207.

[84] Chawla, AS; et al., Optimized image acquisition for breast tomosynthesis in projection and reconstruction space. *Med Phys*, 2009, 36(11), pp. 4859-69.

[85] Lu, Y; et al. Effects of projection-view distributions on image quality of calcifications in digital breast tomosynthesis (DBT) reconstruction., 2010.

[86] Lu, Y; et al., Image quality of microcalcifications in digital breast tomosynthesis: effects of projection-view distributions. *Med Phys*, 2011, 38(10), pp. 5703-12.

[87] Baker, JA; Lo, JY. Breast tomosynthesis: state-of-the-art and review of the literature. *Acad Radiol*, 2011, 18(10), pp. 1298-310.

[88] Brahme, A. *Comprehensive Biomedical Physics*. 2014, Elsevier Science.

[89] Roth, RG. et al., Digital breast tomosynthesis: lessons learned from early clinical implementation. *Radiographics*, 2014, 34(4), pp. E89-102.

[90] Helvie, MA. Digital Mammography Imaging: Breast Tomosynthesis and Advanced Applications. *Radiologic clinics of North America*, 2010, 48(5), pp. 917-929.

[91] Alakhras, M; et al., Digital tomosynthesis: a new future for breast imaging? *Clin Radiol*, 2013, 68(5), pp. e225-36.

[92] Uematsu, T. The emerging role of breast tomosynthesis. *Breast Cancer*, 2013, 20(3), pp. 204-12.

[93] Nguyen, T; et al., Overview of digital breast tomosynthesis: Clinical cases, benefits and disadvantages. *Diagn Interv Imaging*, 2015, 96(9), pp. 843-59.

[94] Viala, J; et al., Stereotactic vacuum-assisted biopsies on a digital breast 3D-tomosynthesis system. *Breast J*, 2013, 19(1), pp. 4-9.

[95] *Breast Tomosynthesis: The Use of Breast Tomosynthesis in a Clinical Setting*, Hologic, Editor., 2015.

[96] Chan, HP; et al., Computer-aided Detection System for Breast Masses on Digital Tomosynthesis Mammograms: Preliminary Experience. *Radiology*, 2005, 237(3), pp. 1075-1080.

[97] Reiser, I; et al., Computerized mass detection for digital breast tomosynthesis directly from the projection images. *Med Phys*, 2006, 33(2), pp. 482-91.

[98] Chan, HP; et al., Computer-aided detection of masses in digital tomosynthesis mammography: comparison of three approaches. *Med Phys*, 2008, 35(9), pp. 4087-95.

[99] Singh, S; et al., Automated breast mass detection in 3D reconstructed tomosynthesis volumes: a featureless approach. *Med Phys*, 2008, 35(8), pp. 3626-36.

[100] Reiser, I; et al., Automated detection of microcalcification clusters for digital breast tomosynthesis using projection data only: a preliminary study. *Med Phys*, 2008, 35(4), pp. 1486-93.

[101] Chen, SC; et al., Initial Clinical Experience with Contrast-Enhanced Digital Breast Tomosynthesis. *Academic radiology*, 2007, 14(2), pp. 229-238.

[102] Puong, S; et al. Optimization of beam parameters and iodine quantification in dual-energy contrast enhanced digital breast tomosynthesis., 2008.

[103] Samei, E; Saunders, RS. Dual-Energy Contrast-Enhanced Breast Tomosynthesis: Optimization of Beam Quality for Dose and Image Quality. *Physics in medicine and biology*, 2011, 56(19), pp. 6359-6378.

[104] Chou, CP; et al., Clinical evaluation of contrast-enhanced digital mammography and contrast enhanced tomosynthesis--Comparison to contrast-enhanced breast MRI. *Eur J Radiol*, 2015, 84(12), pp. 2501-8.

[105] Sinha, SP; et al., Multi-modality 3D breast imaging with X-Ray tomosynthesis and automated ultrasound. *Conf Proc IEEE Eng Med Biol Soc*, 2007, 2007, pp. 1335-8.

[106] Li, J; et al., Effect of a gel retainment dam on automated ultrasound coverage in a dual-modality breast imaging system. *J Ultrasound Med*, 2010, 29(7), pp. 1075-81.

[107] Andersson, I; et al., Breast tomosynthesis and digital mammography: a comparison of breast cancer visibility and BIRADS classification in a population of cancers with subtle mammographic findings. *Eur Radiol*, 2008, 18(12), pp. 2817-25.

[108] Fornvik, D; et al., Breast tomosynthesis: Accuracy of tumor measurement compared with digital mammography and ultrasonography. *Acta Radiol*, 2010, 51(3), pp. 240-7.

[109] Kopans, D; et al., Calcifications in the breast and digital breast tomosynthesis. *Breast J*, 2011, 17(6), pp. 638-44.

[110] Svane, G; et al., Clinical experience of photon counting breast tomosynthesis: comparison with traditional mammography. *Acta Radiol*, 2011, 52(2), pp. 134-42.

[111] Mun, HS; et al., Assessment of extent of breast cancer: comparison between digital breast tomosynthesis and full-field digital mammography. *Clin Radiol*, 2013, 68(12), pp. 1254-9.

[112] Tagliafico, A; et al., Characterisation of microcalcification clusters on 2D digital mammography (FFDM) and digital breast tomosynthesis (DBT): does DBT underestimate microcalcification clusters? Results of a multicentre study. *Eur Radiol*, 2015, 25(1), pp. 9-14.

[113] Skaane, P; et al., Digital breast tomosynthesis (DBT): initial experience in a clinical setting. *Acta Radiol*, 2012, 53(5), pp. 524-9.

[114] Gur, D; et al., Digital breast tomosynthesis: observer performance study. *AJR Am J Roentgenol*, 2009, 193(2), pp.586-91.

[115] Rafferty, EA; et al., Assessing radiologist performance using combined digital mammography and breast tomosynthesis compared with digital mammography alone: results of a multicenter, multireader trial. *Radiology*, 2013, 266(1), pp. 104-13.

[116] McCarthy, AM; et al., Screening Outcomes Following Implementation of Digital Breast Tomosynthesis in a General-Population Screening Program. *Journal of the National Cancer Institute*, 2014, 106(11).

[117] Lourenco, AP; et al., Changes in recall type and patient treatment following implementation of screening digital breast tomosynthesis. *Radiology*, 2015, 274(2), pp. 337-42.

[118] Durand, MA; et al., Early clinical experience with digital breast tomosynthesis for screening mammography. *Radiology*, 2015, 274(1), pp. 85-92.

[119] Spangler, ML; et al., Detection and classification of calcifications on digital breast tomosynthesis and 2D digital mammography: a comparison. *AJR Am J Roentgenol*, 2011, 196(2), pp. 320-4.

[120] Wallis, MG; et al., Two-view and single-view tomosynthesis versus full-field digital mammography: high-resolution X-ray imaging observer study. *Radiology*, 2012, 262(3), pp. 788-96.

[121] Zuley, ML; et al., Comparison of Two-dimensional Synthesized Mammograms versus Original Digital Mammograms Alone and in Combination with Tomosynthesis Images. *Radiology*, 2014, 271(3), pp. 664-671.

[122] Michell, MJ; et al., A comparison of the accuracy of film-screen mammography, full-field digital mammography, and digital breast tomosynthesis. *Clin Radiol*, 2012, 67(10), pp. 976-81.

[123] Good, WF; et al., Digital breast tomosynthesis: a pilot observer study. *AJR Am J Roentgenol*, 2008, 190(4), pp. 865-9.

[124] Astley, S; et al. *A comparison of image interpretation times in full field digital mammography and digital breast tomosynthesis.*, 2013. Proc. SPIE 8673, Medical Imaging 2013: Image Perception, Observer Performance, and Technology Assessment.

[125] *Selenia Dimensions 3D System - P080003/S001.* [cited 2016; Available from: http://www.fda.gov/MedicalDevices/ProductsandMedical Procedures/DeviceApprovalsandClearances/Recently-Approved Devices/ucm353734.htm.

[126] Ciatto, S; et al., Integration of 3D digital mammography with tomosynthesis for population breast-cancer screening (STORM): a prospective comparison study. *Lancet Oncol*, 2013, 14(7), pp. 583-9.

[127] Haas, BM; et al., Comparison of tomosynthesis plus digital mammography and digital mammography alone for breast cancer screening. *Radiology*, 2013, 269(3), pp. 694-700.

[128] Rose, SL; et al., Implementation of breast tomosynthesis in a routine screening practice: an observational study. *AJR Am J Roentgenol*, 2013, 200(6), pp. 1401-8.

[129] Skaane, P; et al., Prospective trial comparing full-field digital mammography (FFDM) versus combined FFDM and tomosynthesis in a population-based screening programme using independent double reading with arbitration. *Eur Radiol*, 2013, 23(8), pp. 2061-71.

[130] Skaane, P; et al., Comparison of digital mammography alone and digital mammography plus tomosynthesis in a population-based screening program. *Radiology*, 2013, 267(1), pp. 47-56.

[131] Skaane, P; et al., Two-view digital breast tomosynthesis screening with synthetically reconstructed projection images: comparison with digital breast tomosynthesis with full-field digital mammographic images. *Radiology*, 2014, 271(3), pp. 655-63.

[132] Friedewald, SM; et al., Breast cancer screening using tomosynthesis in combination with digital mammography. *JAMA*, 2014, 311(24), pp. 2499-2507.

[133] Lang, K; et al., Performance of one-view breast tomosynthesis as a stand-alone breast cancer screening modality: results from the Malmo Breast Tomosynthesis Screening Trial, a population-based study. *Eur Radiol*, 2015.

[134] Gilbert, FJ; et al., The TOMMY trial: a comparison of TOMosynthesis with digital MammographY in the UK NHS Breast Screening Programme--a multicentre retrospective reading study comparing the diagnostic performance of digital breast tomosynthesis and digital mammography with digital mammography alone. *Health Technol Assess*, 2015, 19(4), pp. i-xxv, 1-136.

BIOGRAPHICAL SKETCH

Name: Ana Margarida Mota

Affiliation: Universidade de Lisboa, Faculdade de Ciências, Instituto de Biofísica e Engenharia Biomédica

Education: Integrated Master in Biomedical Engineering

Current PhD student in Biomedical Engineering and Biophysics

Address: Rua Professor Hugo Correia Pardal, 6000-267 Castelo Branco, Portugal (Address for correspondence); Avenida Dom João II, 4.47.01.D, 1990-098 Lisboa, Portugal (Address of residence)

Research and Professional Experience:

Domain of specialization: Medical Imaging is a complex but amazing branch of Biomedical Engineering. It allows us to see what is beyond our eyes. In my opinion, it is one of the most brilliant scientific evolutions in human history because it allows internal structures and physiologic mechanisms to be observed mostly in a non-invasive way.

I have already worked with imaging techniques such as Positron Emission Mammography (master thesis), Image Guided Radiotherapy (in a project at Hospital de Santa Maria), Digital Breast Tomosynthesis (in a national research project) and PET/MRI (in an international research project).

Participation in R&D Projects
Feb 2010 - Dec 2010
Project: Clear-PEM Consortium

Participation: Master Thesis execution "Noise minimization in Positron Emission Mammography images by optimization of acquisition time and voxel size" under orientation of Professor Pedro Almeida and Professor Nuno Matela

Institution: Instituto de Biofísica e Engenharia Biomédica da Faculdade de Ciências da Universidade de Lisboa (Institute of Biophysics and Biomedical Engineering of Faculty of Sciences of Lisbon University)

Oct 2013 – Aug 2014

Project: "Improvement of image quality and dose reduction in digital breast tomosynthesis using statistical image reconstruction algorithms"

Participation: Research Grant in "Development of visualization and optimization methods of image reconstruction algorithms for tomosynthesis" within the unit "UI

645 - 2014," PEst-OE/SAU/UI0645/2014, financed through national funds by FCT under Projects Funding Program of IC&DT Strategic and Public Interest

Institution: Instituto de Biofísica e Engenharia Biomédica da Faculdade de Ciências da Universidade de Lisboa (Institute of Biophysics and Biomedical Engineering of Faculty of Sciences of Lisbon University)

Oct 2014 – Feb 2015

Project: "Establishment of an open database for evaluation of partial volume correction techniques in brain PET/MR studies"

Participation: Visiting Scientist financed through a Short-Term Scientific Mission (STSM) by European Cooperation in Science and Technology and by University College London

Institution: Institute of Nuclear Medicine – University College London/ University College London Hospitals

March 2015 – November 2015

Project: "Improvement of image quality and dose reduction in digital breast tomosynthesis using statistical image reconstruction algorithms"

Participation: Research Grant in "Optimization, validation and integration, in a visualization platform and image analysis previously developed, image reconstruction algorithms developed with IDL and proceed to their clinical evaluation in hospital environment" within the PTDC/BBBIMG/3310/2012, financed through national funds by FCT under Projects Funding Program of IC&DT Strategic and Public Interest

Institution: Instituto de Biofísica e Engenharia Biomédica da Faculdade de Ciências da Universidade de Lisboa (Institute of Biophysics and Biomedical Engineering of Faculty of Sciences of Lisbon University)

Honors:
2003/2004
Honour Distinction with Integration in 2003/2004 Class Excellence of Nuno Álvares Secondary School (merit given since this year to the students who had obtained a final classification greater than 18 (in 20))
Entity: Nuno Álvares Secondary School
2004/2005
Honour Distinction with Integration in 2004/2005 Class Excellence of Nuno Álvares Secondary School
Entity: Nuno Álvares Secondary School

April 2014
3rd Prize obtained in the scientific posters competition with the poster "Improvements on image quality in digital breast tomosynthesis"
Entity: 6th Workshop on Biomedical Engineering
October 2015
Best Student Paper Award
Entity: Conference on Computational Vision and Medical Image Processing: VipIMAGE 2015, Tenerife, Spain
Publications Last 3 Years:
Papers in international scientific periodicals with referees
- A.M. Mota, N. Matela, N. Oliveira, P. Almeida, "Total variation minimization filter for DBT imaging," Medical Physics 42 (6), June 2015. doi: http://dx.doi.org/10.1118/1.4919680.

Papers in conference proceedings
- M. Mota, V. Cuplov, I. Drobnjak, J. Dickson, J. Bert, N. Burgos, J. M. Cardoso, M. Modat, S. Ourselin, J. Schott, K. Erlandsson, B. Hutton and, K. Thielemans, "Establishment of an open database of realistic simulated data for evaluation of partial volume correction techniques in brain PET/MR" EJNMMI Physics 2015, 2(Suppl 1): A44 La Biodola, Isola d'Elba, Italy, May 2015. doi: 10.1186/2197-7364-2-S1-A44.
- M. Mota, N. Matela, N. Oliveira and P. Almeida, "An iterative algorithm for Total Variation minimization in DBT imaging" Proceedings of the V ECCOMAS Thematic Conference on Computational Vision and Medical Image Processing: VipIMAGE 2015, Tenerife, Spain, October 2015.

Posters in conferences

- M. Mota, N. Matela and N. Oliveira. "Improvements on image quality in digital breast tomosynthesis." In 6th Workshop on Biomedical Engineering. Lisboa, Portugal, 2014.
- A M. Mota, V. Cuplov, I. Drobnjak, J. Dickson, J. Bert, N. Burgos, J. M. Cardoso, M. Modat, S. Ourselin, J. Schott, K. Erlandsson, B. Hutton and, K. Thielemans, "Establishment of an open database of realistic simulated data for evaluation of partial volume correction techniques in brain PET/MR," in PSMR 2015: 4th Conference on PET/MR and SPECT/MR, Isola d'Elba, Italy, May 2015.

Oral communications in conferences

- M. Mota, N. Matela, N. Oliveira and P. Almeida, "An iterative algorithm for Total Variation minimization in DBT imaging," Conference on Computational Vision and Medical Image Processing: VipIMAGE 2015, Tenerife, Spain, October 2015.

For more information, please go to http://ibeb.fc.ul.pt/ana-mota/.

In: Digital Tomosynthesis
Editor: Lucia Gutierrez

ISBN: 978-1-63485-132-9
© 2016 Nova Science Publishers, Inc.

Chapter 3

SYSTEM OPTIMIZATION: IMAGE RECONSTRUCTION AND IMAGING CONFIGURATION OPTIMIZATION WITH A MULTI-BEAM PARALLEL DIGITAL BREAST TOMOSYNTHESIS SYSTEM

Sasi K. Allada[1], BS, Rajamohan R. Kalluru[2], PhD, Tom Rishel[1], MS, and Weihua Zhou[1], PhD
[1]Department of Computer Science,
[2]Department of Physics and Astronomy,
University of Southern Mississippi, MS, US

ABSTRACT

Digital breast tomosynthesis is a novel technology that provides 3D information of the breast and helps to identify the malignant cancer tissue from overlying healthy breast tissue. Optimizing image reconstruction and imaging configuration of a multi-beam parallel digital breast tomosynthesis system is in demand. Numerously used algorithms from the typical image reconstruction models which are used for iso-centric tomosynthesis systems were investigated for the present multi-beam parallel tomosynthesis imaging system. The representative algorithms, including back-projection (BP), filtered back-projection (FBP), matrix inversion tomosynthesis reconstruction (MITS), maximum likelihood expectation maximization (MLEM), ordered-subset maximum likelihood expectation maximization (OS-MLEM), and simultaneous algebraic reconstruction technique (SART), were implemented to fit our system design. Experiments, based on phantoms and computer simulations, illustrate that the prototype system combined with developed algorithms is capable of providing three-dimensional information of the objects with good image quality and has abilities to improve digital breast tomosynthesis technology.

Four methodologies were employed to optimize the reconstruction algorithms and different imaging configurations were tested for the prototype system. A linear tomosynthesis imaging analysis tool was used to investigate blurring-out reconstruction algorithms. Computer simulations of sphere and wire objects were used to evaluate the performance of various out-of-plane artifact removal approaches. A frequency-domain-based methodology, relative NEQ(f) analysis, was investigated to evaluate the overall system performance based on the propagation of signal and noise. This study had three over all findings: the iterative reconstruction algorithms remove more out-of-plane blur; increasing the view angle could decrease out-of-plane blur; and increasing the number of projection images can improve the in-focus sharpness of the objects.

1. INTRODUCTION

Digital Breast Tomosynthesis (DBT), an emerging and improving breast imaging technology, enhances the diagnosis of early breast cancer by providing in-depth information about the overlapping dense breast tissues with no ambiguities. It promises to reduce recall rates, enhance the biopsy choice of patients, and increase cancer detection accuracy (Park et al. 2007).

The typical breast tomosynthesis prototype systems acquire projection images with the X-ray tube moving along an arc path. This kind of implementation can reutilize the traditional mammography design, decrease the cost and reduce the training procedure for the operators. However, the X-ray tube's movement may introduce motion blur to tomosynthesis images as well as cause patient discomfort.

A novel nanotechnology enabled X-ray source, invented by Zhou et al. has been investigated for DBT applications (Yang et al. 2008, Zhou et al. 2010, Balla et al. 2010, Rayford et al. 2013, Zhou et al. 2015a, Zhou et al. 2015b). This system provides two important advantages in terms of imaging. First, X-ray generation can be rapidly turned on or off, thus reducing the motional blurring and providing enhanced resolution. Second, this system can generate tomographic images without moving the patient or the X-ray source. This provides enormous advantages in terms of image acquisition speed and image quality (Juliano et al. 2011).

2. Current State of Digital Breast Tomosynthesis

2.1. System Design of Digital Breast Tomosynthesis Imaging Systems

A typical tomosynthesis imaging system can be decomposed into three parts: image acquisition, image reconstruction and image display.

The tomosynthesis reconstruction is implemented on a computer with high performance computation. The body component or volume is divided into small voxels, and each voxel represents one element with unique homogeneous intensity. The intensity of every voxel is solved based on the reconstruction model. The reconstruction results are sent to the display to be checked by the radiologists. Some functions, including image contrast enhancement and marking, may be provided. The efficacy of DBT depends on the image quality. High DQE detectors, imaging configuration, an accurate reconstruction algorithm, and high-definition image monitor, for example, contribute to high image quality.

A. Imaging Geometry of Current DBT Systems

The current DBT systems re-utilize the conventional mammography design called the partial iso-centric design where the breast object is located above the detector surface with compression. Figure 1 shows the schematic of a typical partial iso-centric digital tomosynthesis system design. An X-ray tube moves above the breast object to specified positions with the limited angle access to acquire the dataset of projection images.

B. Imaging Geometry of a Novel Multi-Beam Parallel DBT Prototype System

A prototype system, fixed multi-beam field emission tomosynthesis imaging with parallel imaging geometry has been invented and developed to eliminate the motion blur due to the X-ray tube motion associated with partial iso-centric design of typical DBT prototype systems (Lalush et al. 2006; Yang et al. 2008). Moreover, the image acquisition speed is faster when compared with the other designs.

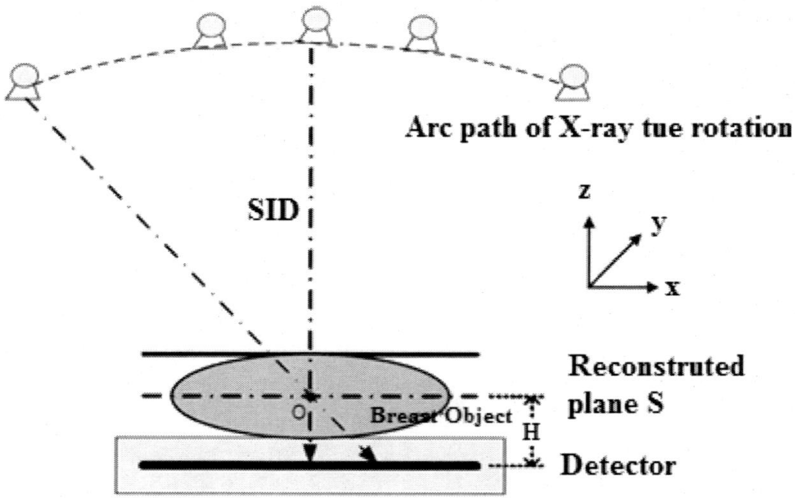

Figure 1. Imaging geometry of the partial iso-centric DBT systems.

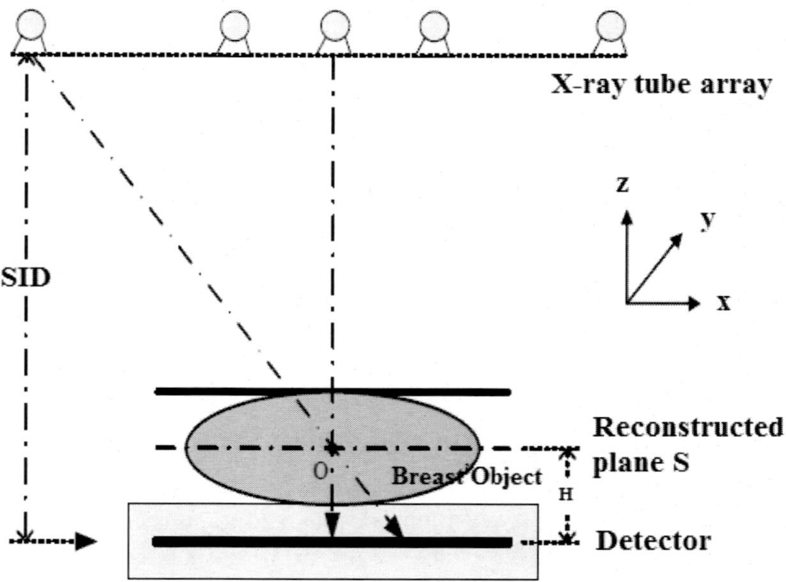

Figure 2. Imaging geometry of the multi-beam parallel DBT system.

The new parallel tomosynthesis imaging configuration is illustrated in Figure 2. Multiple X-ray sources are fixed along a line, parallel to the detector to avoid the X-ray tube's motion. Control signals are triggered to activate each X-ray tube sequentially to acquire a complete dataset of tomosynthesis projections.

2.2. Technical Evaluation of Image Quality of DBT Systems

Both the blur and noise of images influence the visibility of objects and are major barriers to accurate identification of the actual objects on the images. The artifacts may be mistakenly interpreted and create images which do not represent the body structure. A good image should provide an accurate representation of the size, shape and relative position of objects.

A good trade-off has to be carefully kept in adjusting imaging variables to maximize object visibility, in most cases, because a change in one variable may adversely affect the other image quality evaluation factors, such as radiation exposure (Sprawls 1998).

In the spatial domain, image quality can be quantified by the signal to noise ratio (SNR) and contrast to noise ratio (CNR). A high value of each of these parameters means a better imaging system, but often compromises among the parameters have to be made. On the other hand, in the frequency domain, modulation transfer function (MTF), noise power spectrum (NPS) and noise equivalent quanta (NEQ) are used repeatedly to characterize the performance of imaging systems and digital detectors. Physical measurements and computational analysis of MTF, NPS and NEQ are well known (Dobbins 2000; Samei et al. 2006; Dobbins et al. 2006; Chen al 2007b; Zhou et al. 2013).

3. IMAGE RECONSTRUCTION ALGORITHMS FOR A MULTI-BEAM PARALLEL DBT SYSTEM

The tomosynthesis reconstruction algorithms translate two-dimensional projection images into three-dimensional slice images. Tomosynthesis imaging in the early stage used a shift-and-add (SAA) reconstruction algorithm, which provided limited image quality due to out-of-plane blurring (Niklason et al. 1997, Chen et al. 2007a). The other reconstruction algorithm, called back-projection (BP), was developed in order to reduce the out-of-plane blurring

(Chen et al. 2007a). Filters were added to BP to reduce noise and improve the conspicuity of objects, which formed the filtered back-projection method (FBP). Currently, FBP is one of the most commonly used reconstruction methods (Matsuo et al. 1993, Lauritsch and Haerer 1998, Cong et al. 2011).

The blurring functions were proposed to solve the out-of-plane problems generated by the planes immediately adjacent to the plane of interest (Ghosh Roy et al. 1985). An extended blur function could be used to find the exact solution of in-plane structures from a complete set of tomosynthesized planes (Dobbins et al. 1987, Dobbins 1990).

When the reconstructed object is divided into a great number of small non-overlapping voxels with constant attenuation coefficients, the other perspective can be proposed to explain the reconstructed images. Firstly, the Beer-Lambert Law tells us

$$T = I \cdot e^{-ul} \tag{Eq. 1}$$

where T is the transmitted X-ray intensity, I is the incident X-ray intensity, u is the attenuation coefficient, and l is the length of the path where the X-ray projection line passes through the voxel. The pixel value on the reconstruction image represents the attenuation coefficient for the tomosynthesis imaging process.

To obtain the attenuation coefficients, one method is to employ the maximum likelihood model, which maximizes the probability of acquiring the measured projections from the incident X-ray and the current imaging parameters (Lange and Carson, 1984; Lange and Fessler 1995). Wu et al. used maximum likelihood expectation maximization (MLEM) in a partial iso-centric DBT prototype system and compared it with BP and FBP (Wu et al. 2003, 2004). Their results suggested that BP provided the best SDNR for low-contrast masses but limited conspicuity; FBP provided the high edge sharpness for micro-calcifications, but the image quality of masses was poor; the information of both the masses and the micro-calcification were well restored with balanced quality by the MLEM algorithm (Wu et al. 2004).

Alternatively, the attenuation coefficients could be obtained by using algebraic reconstruction techniques (Andersen and Kak, 1984; Andersen, 1989), which iteratively generates a new set of projection images from the estimate of the coefficients, compares the simulated images to real projection data, smears the difference back to generate a new estimate of coefficients, and thus provides a solution of the attenuation coefficients. Zhang et al. used the simultaneous algebraic reconstruction technique (SART) in a partial iso-centric DBT prototype system and compared it with BP and MLEM (Zhang et al. 2006). Their results suggested that the BP method provided very smooth reconstructed images with low background noise, while the SART and MLEM methods considerably enhanced the contrast and edges of the features but simultaneously amplified the image noise; the BP method had blurring artifacts in the X-ray source motion direction that obscured the contrast-detail objects, while the other two methods could significantly improve object conspicuity.

3.1. Back Projection (BP)

The BP algorithm, similar to the SAA algorithm, is a common mathematic reconstruction algorithm (Chen et al. 2007a, Chen et al. 2010). Unlike the SAA algorithm, the BP algorithm calculates the shift amount along both the x and y directions for each pixel on the reconstruction plane in order to improve the reconstruction of the single pixel on a reconstruction plane at some certain height above the detector (Zhou et al. 2014). Figure 3 illustrates the BP reconstruction for a multi-beam parallel DBT system. $A(A_x,A_y,A_z)$ represents the coordinate of the object on the reconstruction plane R. $B(B_x,B_y,B_z)$ represents the projection coordinate of the point A on the detector plane. $R(R_x,R_y,R_z)$ represents the coordinate of the X-ray source R. A's pixel value can be found by referring to its projected point B. The location relationship can be written as

$$B_x = R_x + \frac{R_z}{R_z - A_z} \cdot (A_x - R_x)$$

$$B_y = R_y + \frac{R_z}{R_z - A_z} \cdot (A_y - R_y)$$

(Eq. 2)

The final pixel value of the point A in the BP reconstruction is calculated by the following

$$S = \frac{1}{N} \sum_{i=1}^{N} I(B_i)$$

(Eq. 3)

where $I(B_i)$ is the back projected pixel value based on Eq. 2 for the pixel A and the ith projection image (X-ray source), and N is the total number of projection images.

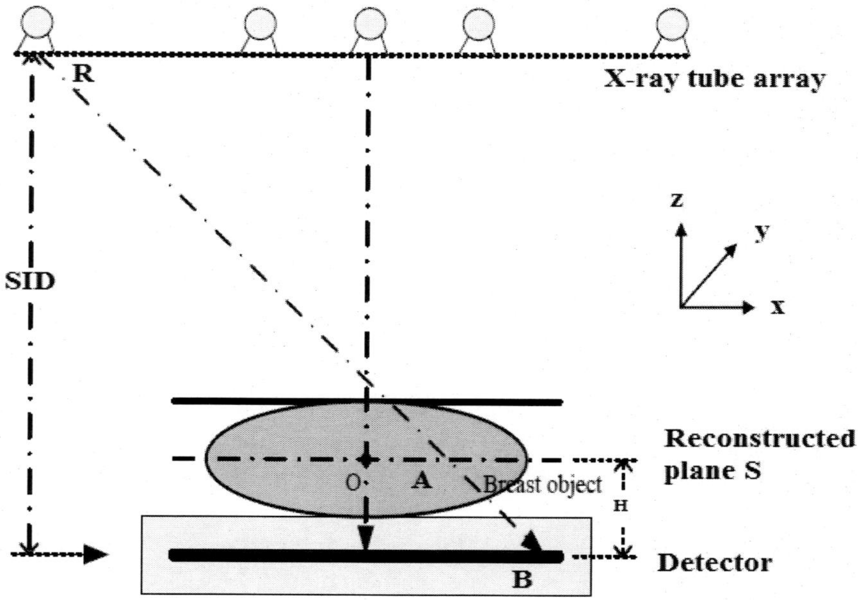

Figure 3. BP reconstruction for a multi-beam parallel DBT system.

3.2. Filtered Back-Projection (FBP)

The FBP algorithms (Stevens et al. 2001, Mertelemeier et al. 2006) model the projection and back projection based on Radon transform and Fourier slice theorem and has been a classic family of reconstruction algorithms for X-ray imaging.

3.2.1. Radon Transform

Radon transform (Radon 1917, Gonzalez and Woods, 2008) presents the integral relationship between the original object and its projection. It can be written as

$$g(s,\theta) = \int\limits_{-\infty}^{+\infty} \int\limits_{-\infty}^{+\infty} f(x,y)\delta(x\cos\theta + y\sin\theta - s)dxdy$$

(Eq. 4)

where x, y, s and θ are variables. δ is an impulse function. $f(x, y)$ is the object function and $g(s,\theta)$ is the projection function.

Changing the variables with respect to a fixed variable and so forth yields another projection. By summing up Radon projections along all angles passing the same pixel, the back projection is as following:

$$\tilde{f}(x,y) = \int\limits_{0}^{\pi} g(x\cos\theta + y\sin\theta, \theta)$$

(Eq. 5)

$\tilde{f}(x,y)$ is an approximation of the image from which the projection is generated.

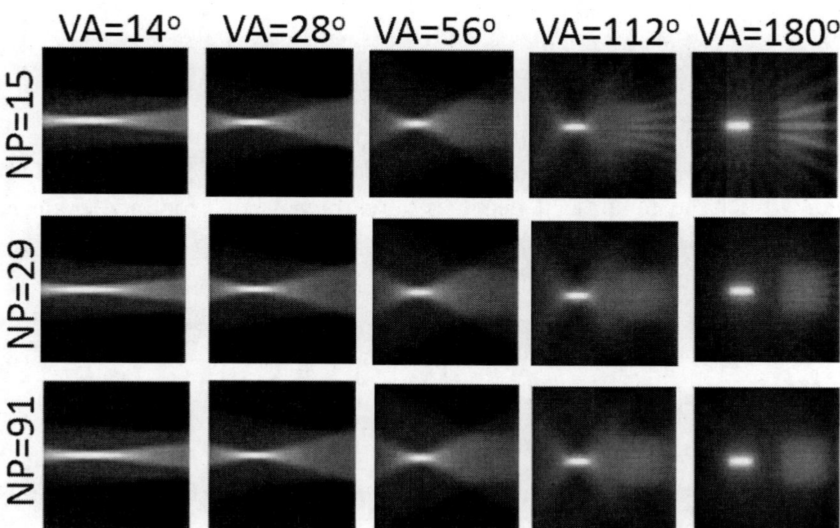

Figure 4. Image reconstruction by inverse Radon transform.

The sampling rates have a profound influence on image reconstruction results. Figure 4 shows the image reconstruction results by inverse Radon transform in terms of increased view angle (VA) versus number of projection images (NP). The increased VA/NP numbers reveal the reconstructed image structures of the object with shaper edges and less blur.

3.2.2. Filtered Back Projection (FBP)

The Fourier-slice theorem (Gonzalez and Woods, 2008) depicts that the Fourier Transform of a projection is a slice of the 2D Fourier Transform of the region from which the projection is obtained. The 2D inverse Fourier transform of $F(u,v)$ is the following

$$f(x,y)) = \int_{-\infty}^{+\infty} \int_{-\infty}^{+\infty} F(u,v)e^{j2\pi\omega(ux+vy)}\,du\,dv$$

(Eq. 6)

In polar coordinates, if we let $u = \omega\cos\theta$ and $v = \omega\sin\theta$, the equation becomes

$$f(x,y)) = \int_{0}^{\pi} \left[\int_{-\infty}^{+\infty} |\omega|G(\omega,\theta)e^{j2\pi\omega\rho}\,d\omega \right]_{\rho=x\cos\theta+y\sin\theta} d\theta$$

(Eq. 7)

The inverse Fourier Transform is undefined for the ramp filter $|\omega|$ as its amplitude extends to infinity in both directions. In practice, the method is to window/filter the ramp so it becomes zeros outside of a defined frequency interval (Gonzalez and Woods, 2008).

The following filters were used in our FBP reconstruction (Zhou 2012):

Ramp filter: The Ramp filter reflects the sampling geometry of the scanning process. It is designed based on the sampling density as follows:

$$H_{Ramp}(\omega_x,\omega_y,\omega_z) = \sqrt{\omega_x^2 + \omega_z^2}$$

(Eq. 8)

where ω is the frequency bin.

Han filter: The Han filter is used to change the frequency response of ramp-filtered BP reconstruction. With realistic noisy data, it can also smooth the image. It can be written as:

$$H_{Han} = 0.5\left(1 + \cos\left(\frac{\pi\omega_x}{\omega_N}\right)\right)$$

(Eq. 9)

where ω_N is the total frequency bin number in the x direction.

Gaussian filter: In order to control the high frequency noise amplification in FBP, a Gaussian filter is also applied:

$$H_{Gaussian} = e^{-\frac{u^2}{k^2}}$$

(Eq. 10)

where u is the individual frequency bin and k is the kernel size. $k = 30$ is used in our experiments.

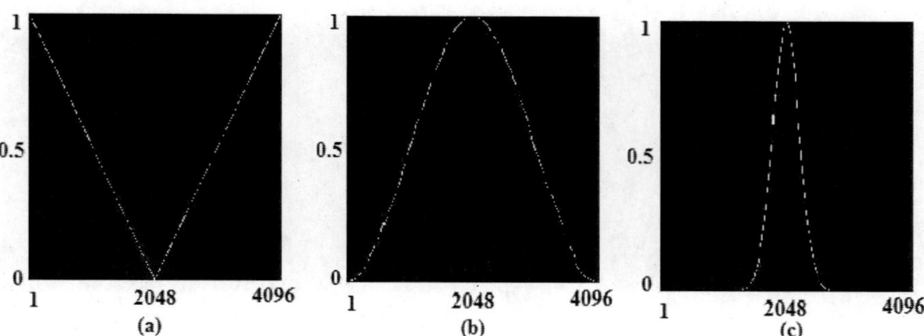

Figure 5. Filters used in the FBP reconstruction. (a) Ramp filter. (b) Han filter. (c) Gaussian filter. Horizontal axis, frequency bin; vertical axis, normalized frequency.

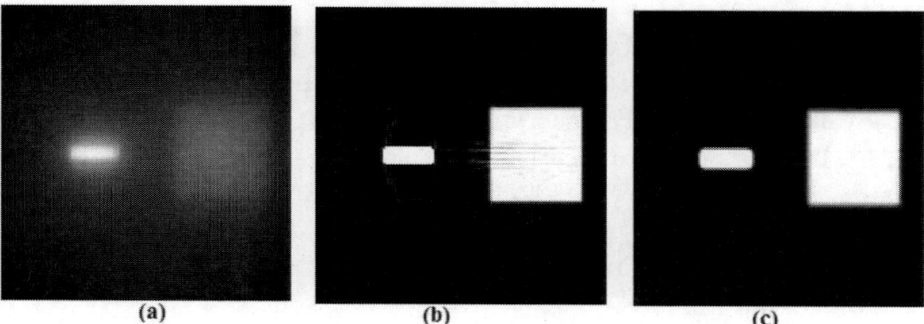

Figure 6. 2D images reconstructed by FBP. (a) Without any filter (only inverse Radon transform applied). (b) With the Ramp filter. (c) With the Ramp and Han filter.

Figure 5 shows the shapes of these three filters. Figure 6 compares the reconstructed results with different filter settings. The blur artifact in Figure 6a is minimized with the ramp filter, as shown in Figure 6b. Further use of the Han filter suppresses the ring artifact and the final reconstructed image is shown in Figure 6c.

3.3. Matrix Inversion Tomosynthesis (MITS)

The use of linear algebra in MITS is a good solution for the relative blur in each reconstructed plane (Dobbins et al. 1987, Dobbins 1990, Godfrey et al. 2006). If the structures in the ith plane are defined as p_i then the tomosynthesized images s_i can be described as

$$s_1 = p_1 \otimes f_{11} + p_2 \otimes f_{12} + \ldots\ldots + p_n \otimes f_{1n}$$
$$s_2 = p_2 \otimes f_{21} + p_2 \otimes f_{22} + \ldots\ldots + p_n \otimes f_{2n}$$
$$\ldots\ldots$$
$$s_n = p_1 \otimes f_{n1} + p_2 \otimes f_{n2} + \ldots\ldots + p_n \otimes f_{nn} \qquad \text{(Eq. 11)}$$

where f_{ij} is the blurring function for the structures in the plane j that appear in the tomosynthesized image of the plane i. The convolutions of the above equations become simply multiplications in Fourier space. In matrix form, it will be

$$S = M \times P \qquad \text{(Eq. 12)}$$

where M is the matrix of Fourier Transforms of blurring functions.

By multiplying each side of the equation by the inverse of the matrix M, the patient structure P in Frequency space can be acquired. Then by taking the inverse Fourier transform, we can get the patient structure

$$P = M^{-1} \times S \qquad \text{(Eq. 13)}$$

3.4. Maximum Likelihood Expectation Maximization (MLEM) and Ordered Subset - Maximum Likelihood Expectation Maximization (OS-MLEM)

Statistical reconstruction attempts to maximize the likelihood of getting the detected X-ray intensity from the incident intensity and X-ray attenuation model. MLEM to acquire the attenuation coefficients u can be written as (Wu et al. 2003, Wu et al. 2004):

$$u_j^{(t+1)} = u_j^{(t)} + \Delta u_j^{(t)} = u_j^{(t)} + \frac{u_j^{(t)} \sum_i l_{ij}\left(I_i\, e^{-<l,u^{(t)}>_i} - T_i\right)}{\sum_i \left(l_{ij} <l,u^{(t)}>_i\, I_i\, e^{-<l,u^{(t)}>_i}\right)} \qquad \text{(Eq. 14)}$$

$$<l,u>_i = \sum_i l_{ij} u_j$$

where T_i is the transmitted X-ray intensity or detected pixel value on the detector for the X-ray projection line i. j is the individual voxel in the three-dimensional attenuation model. $<l, u>_i$ means the total attenuation of the X-ray projection line i. I_i is the incident X-ray intensity to pixel i. Usually, we can replace I_i with the flat image. l_{ij} is the path length of the intersection between the voxel j and the X-ray projection line from the X-ray source to the pixel i on the detector.

Reducing the loop complexity in standard MLEM implementations will improve the computational efficiency. It is possible to reduce the loop complexity by introducing a simplified and equivalent implementation with a novel data structure for the ray-tracing method.

MLEM Acceleration Using the Sparse-Matrix-Based Method (Zhou et al. 2008)

The ray tracing technique is a frequently used method to solve the length of the path where each X-ray projection line passes through each voxel (Chen 2007c, Zhou 2015b). In fact, on every reconstruction plane, for each X-ray projection line i, only a few voxels are perorated. This results in a sparse matrix condition. The sparse matrix is involved in the strategy of managing the relationship between the X-ray projection line i, the voxel j, and the path length l_{ij}. The combination of an array and linked lists is adopted here. The algorithm utilizes the feature of the sparse matrix to reduce the allocated memory for the calculation of the path l_{ij} as it is convenient to traverse the voxels which are penetrated by the X-ray projection line i. This linked list based on the sparse matrix serves as the foundation of the loop order adjustment. The time complexity decreases from $O(t*j*i^2)$ to $O(t*i*\eta)$ for the accelerated MLEM algorithm, when η is not greater than the maximum number of the voxels associated with X-ray projection line i ($\eta<<j$). Compared to the standard MLEM implementation, the accelerated MLEM implementation is capable of producing the same image quality with a much faster running speed.

Ordered Subset - Maximum Likelihood Expectation Maximization (OS-MLEM)

The OS-MLEM algorithm has gained substantial interest for tomosynthesis image reconstruction due to its acceleration of the MLEM algorithm. It has the following advantages (Erdogan et al. 1999):

a. OS-MLEM provides an order-of-magnitude acceleration over MLEM. In OS-MLEM, only a subset of the projection image dataset is used for each iteration.
b. Good image quality can be acquired.
c. OS-MLEM is easily implemented with slight modification of the MLEM algorithm.

However, because OS-MLEM uses part of the projection views when updating the attenuation coefficients, it is not stable when reaching convergence. To improve the convergence, the special update order was designed to maximize the angle separation between the successive absorbed projection views (Li et al. 1993).

3.5. Simultaneous Algebraic Reconstruction Technique (SART)

The algebraic reconstruction technique iteratively generates a new set of projection images from the estimate of attenuation coefficients, compares the simulated images to real projection data and then smears the difference back to generate a new estimate of attenuation coefficients. After the iterations, the attenuation coefficients are obtained. The following is the SART algorithm for the estimation of the attenuation coefficients u (Zhang et al. 2006):

$$u_j^{(t+1)} = u_j^{(t)} + \Delta u_j^{(t)} = u_j^{(t)} + \frac{\sum_i l_{ij} \left(\dfrac{D_i - \sum_j l_{ij} u_j^t}{\sum_i l_{ij}} \right)}{\sum_i l_{i,j}}$$

(Eq. 15)

where $D_i = \log \dfrac{I_i}{T_i}$

4. OPTIMIZATION OF IMAGE RECONSTRUCTION AND IMAGING CONFIGURATION FOR A MULTI-BEAM PARALLEL DIGITAL BREAST TOMOSYNTHESIS SYSTEM

One key objective in digital tomosynthesis imaging is the optimization of various tomosynthesis reconstruction algorithms. The variable configurable parameters should also be optimized to improve the system performance. Four methodologies have been developed to optimize the design of the new multi-beam parallel DBT system (Zhou 2012).

4.1. Linear Tomosynthesis Imaging Analysis

In tomosynthesis reconstruction, reconstruction slices passing through an object are reconstructed based on a tomosynthesis dataset of X-ray projection images. Digital computers are usually used to compute the reconstruction so it is necessary to represent the actual continuous object as a discrete set of numbers, such as pixels or voxels.

Ignoring the statistical nature of the imaging process, the mapping from the object o to a single projection image p can be written as (Barrett et al. 2004):

$$p = h \times o$$

(Eq. 16)

The mapping operator h can be either linear or nonlinear. The property of homogeneity in linear systems makes it easier to analyze than nonlinear ones.

Here we begin with the assumption of linearity. In Fourier frequency domain, one can use

$$P = H \times O \qquad \text{(Eq. 17)}$$

to denote the imaging mapping. H is the Fourier transform of h and it represents the transfer function. P and O are the Fourier representations of the projection image p and the object o, respectively.

For a linear tomosynthesis imaging configuration with N evenly distributed X-ray sources of parallel imaging configurations, the impulse response is simply a series of N infinitesimal points. The corresponding transfer function is extended into (Grant 1972):

$$H^N\left(w_x \mid Z\right) = \frac{1}{N} \frac{\sin N\left(\frac{\delta w_x}{2}\right)}{\sin\left(\frac{\delta w_x}{2}\right)} \qquad \text{(Eq. 18)}$$

where H is the transfer function, Z is the depth, w_x is spatial frequency conjugate to x, δ is the impulse function.

The transfer function is a direct quantitative measure of the system's ability to blur undesirable planes and it provides a valid method of comparing imaging configurations.

The application of linear tomosynthesis imaging theory (Godfrey et al. 2006, Zhou 2012) to analyze the multi-beam digital breast tomosynthesis system brings the following suggestions:

a. Out-of-plane objects will be better suppressed as the number of projection images increase.
b. For the same number of projection images, if view angle increases, denser contours appear.

The dense contour decreases with the increase of the sampling frequency in slice thickness. This means that when reducing the slice thickness, the out-of-plane artifacts will be better reduced.

Linear analysis of tomosynthesis imaging configurations provides a practical tool to optimize the system design, however it has some limitations because many detectors and reconstruction algorithms are inherently nonlinear.

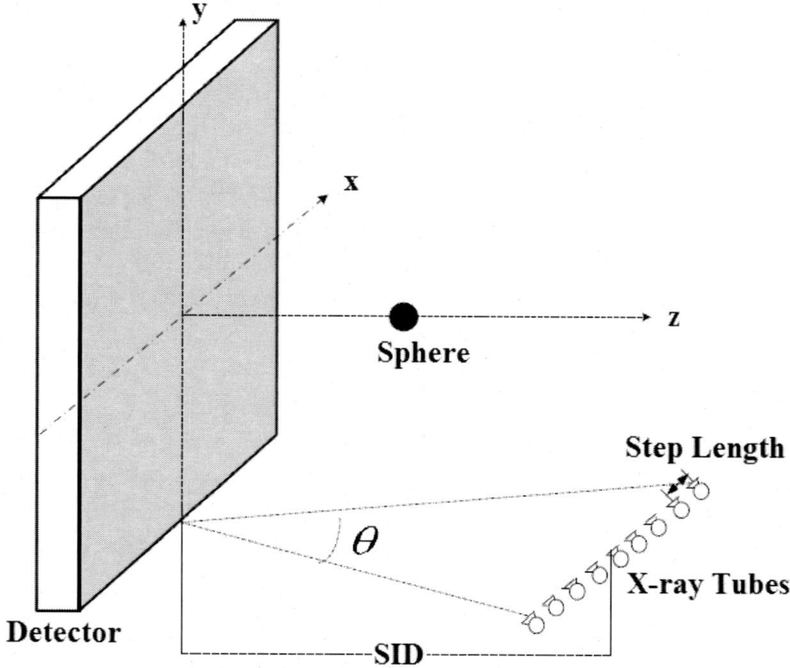

Figure 7. Sphere imaging simulation.

4.2. Sphere Simulation

The sphere simulation was designed to evaluate the removal of out-of-plane artifacts with different imaging configurations and reconstruction algorithms (Chen et al. 2009, Zhou 2012). A spherical object, placed at the center of a plane with the height of 20 mm above the detector, was simulated and embedded in a non-uniform background as the target to evaluate the imaging configurations and reconstruction algorithms. The linear attenuation coefficient of the simulated spherical object was set to 0.038 /mm, which referred to the linear attenuation coefficient of carcinoma tissue for 30 KeV photon energy (Guimarães et al. 2009). The ray-tracing method was used to calculate the X-ray attenuation. Figure 7 illustrates the imaging simulation. The X-ray tubes were placed horizontally, and the horizontal blur dominates the blur of the reconstructed planes, so the horizontal axis dominated the out-of-plane artifacts and the line profiles through the center of the sphere along the horizontal axis were extracted to evaluate the out-of-plane blur and in-focus peak sharpness.

Five representative algorithms, including BP, FBP, MITS, MLEM and SART were applied to reconstruct 3D information of the simulated objects. For in-focus sharpness analysis, FBP, MITS and SART algorithms showed the edge enhancement, as illustrated by solid line profiles from FPB reconstructed spheres in Figure 8. The edge enhancement also exists for the partial iso-centric tomosynthesis imaging configuration, which is common for current breast tomosynthesis systems. For out-of-plane blur analysis, the big view angle reduced the out-of-plane blur, as illustrated by the dotted line profiles in Figure 8.

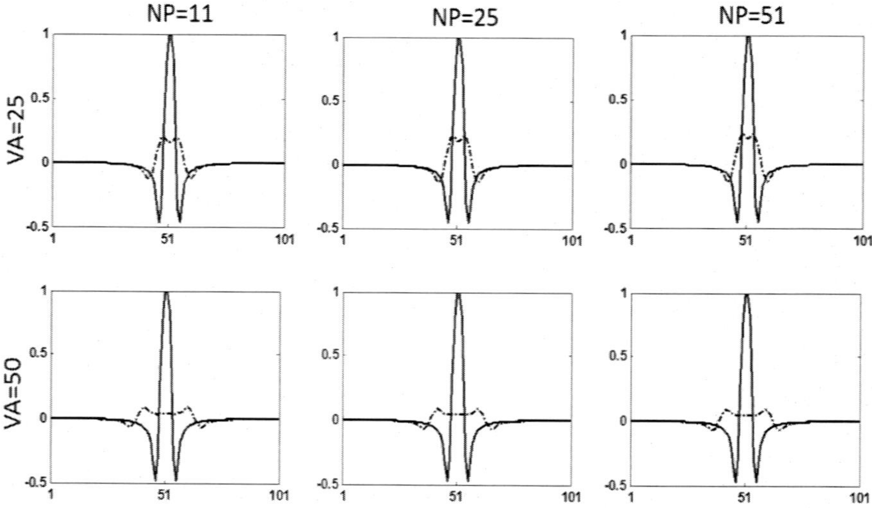

Figure 8. Line profiles at FBP reconstructed spheres. Solid lines were extracted from the plane 20mm above the detector. Dotted lines were extracted from the plane 23mm above the detector.

4.3. Wire Simulation

The wire simulation was designed to evaluate the reconstruction algorithms and imaging configurations based on the impulse response characterization (Balla et al. 2010, Zhou 2012). The experiments referred to the method of optimizing the chest tomosynthesis system by Godfrey et al. (Godfrey et al. 2006). To evaluate the combinations of VA and NP, 11, 25 and

51 projection images of a very thin wire running vertically through the image space, whose depth varied from z = 30 mm to z = 60 mm from the bottom to top were simulated. Figure 9 shows the geometry of the wire simulation. Each point on the simulated wire was considered as an impulse. Simulated acquisition allowed the generation of noise-free projection images that contained only a single impulse for each column in the image.

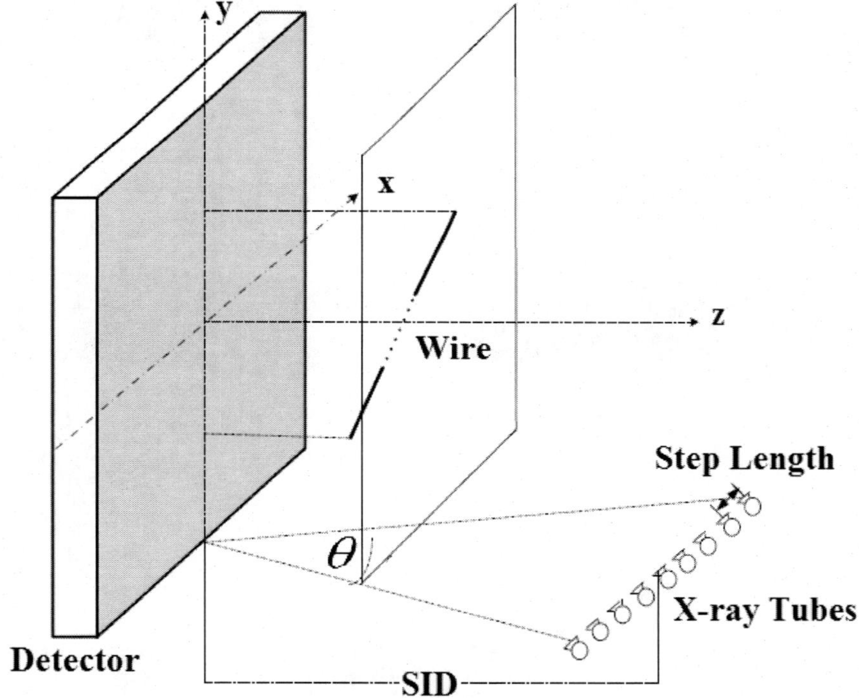

Figure 9. Wire imaging simulation.

Five representative algorithms, including BP, FBP, MITS, MLEM and SART were applied to reconstruct the wire. When the number of projection images increased, the conspicuity of the in-plane point along the simulated wire became stronger. Compared to other reconstruction algorithms, MLEM showed better performance in removing the out-of-plane blur (Figure 10).

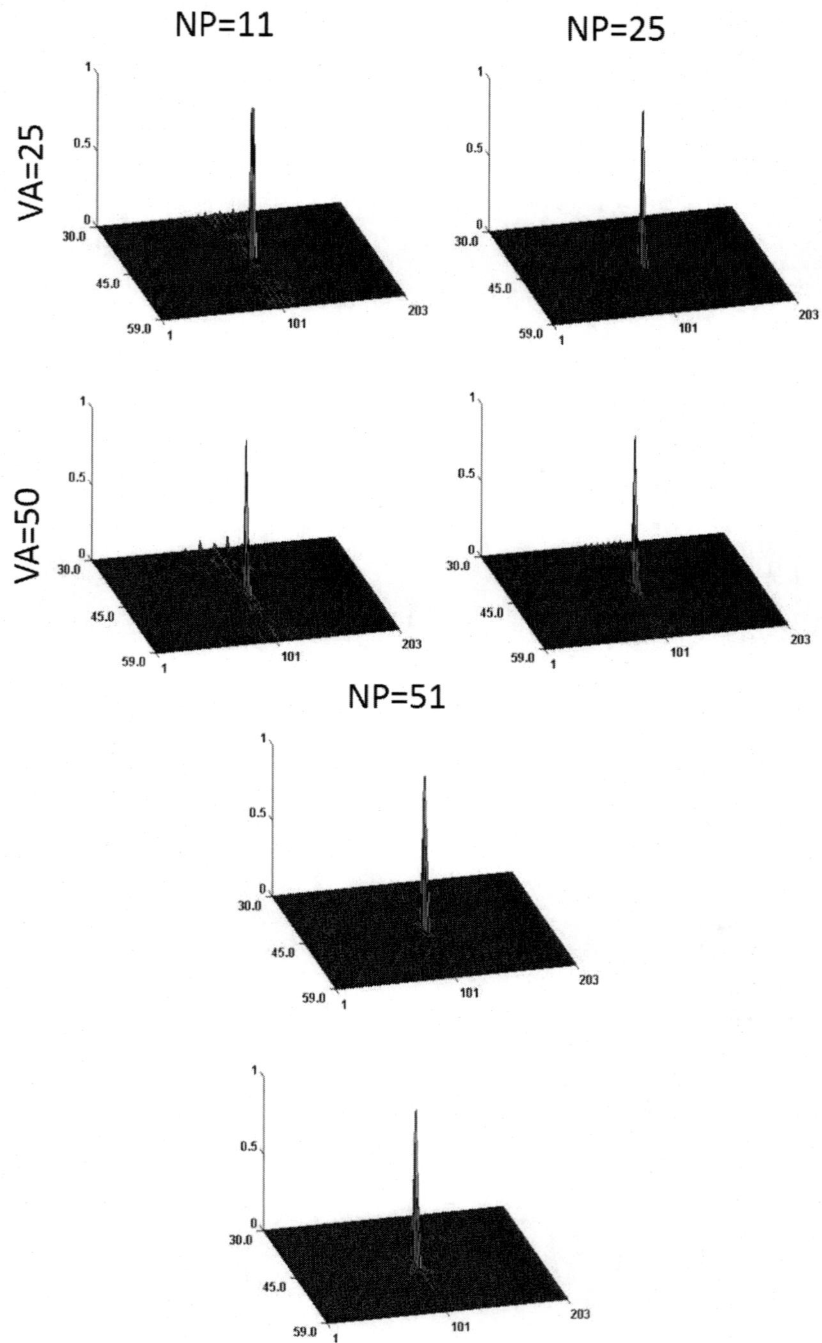

Figure 10. Impulse responses of wire simulation with MLEM reconstruction.

5. RELATIVE NEQ (f) ANALYSIS OF A MULTI-BEAM PARALLEL DIGITAL BREAST TOMOSYNTHESIS SYSTEM

The noise-equivalent quanta NEQ (f) describes the minimum number of X-ray quanta required to produce a specified signal to noise ratio (SNR) (Dobbins and Godfrey 2003). NEQ(f) has been accepted as the measurement metric of medical imaging systems as it describes how well a low-contrast structure can be detected in a uniform noise-limited image by the ideal observer. It is dependent on the overall system performance, including the radiation dosage, imaging configuration, pulse width, detector and image reconstruction algorithm. The NEQ(f) is the ratio of modulation transfer function (MTF(f)) and noise power spectrum (NPS(f)).

The investigated digital breast tomosynthesis system has 29 X-ray beam sources. A digital flat-panel detector with the pixel pitch of 140μm was integrated into the prototype system. The image size was 2048×1664. Two imaging configuration modes were used: (1) view angle = 14 degrees, number of projection images = 15 (Mode code: VA14NP15); (2) view angle = 28 degrees, number of projection images = 15 (Mode code: VA28NP15).

5.1. Modulation Transfer Function (MTF)

The *MTF(f)* analyzes the resolution of imaging system in frequency domain. The composite *MTF(f)* of a tomosynthesis imaging system is the product of the MTFs coming from all individual stages including both image acquisition MTF (*MTFproj(f)*) and image reconstruction MTF (*MTFrecon(f)*).

5.1.1. Projection MTF(f)

Two methods, slit method and edge method, are recommended for breast tomosynthesis systems (Dobbins 2000). The MTFproj(f) of our breast tomosynthesis prototype system was tested with a slit method (Fujita et al. 1992) that was applied to measure the presampling MTF's of a computed radiographic system. The experiments, the results by Qian et al. (Qian et al. 2012) were used.

5.1.2. Reconstruction MTF(f)

The *MTFrecon(f)* presents the spatial frequency response with respect to different imaging configurations and reconstruction algorithms. The

MTFrecon(f) can be calculated as the Fourier Transform of the impulse response along the tube's alignment direction. Figure 11 illustrates the imaging simulation. The *MTFrecon(f)* varies with the location of the simulated impulse. In our experiments, two areas were computer simulated with the imaging configurations of the prototype systems: the first area, "away-from-chest-wall," was used to mimic an object away from the chest wall; the second area, "near-chest-wall," was used to mimic an object near chest wall. In each area, 25 impulses were evenly placed inside the pixel. The ray-tracing method was used to generate the projection images and then reconstructed.

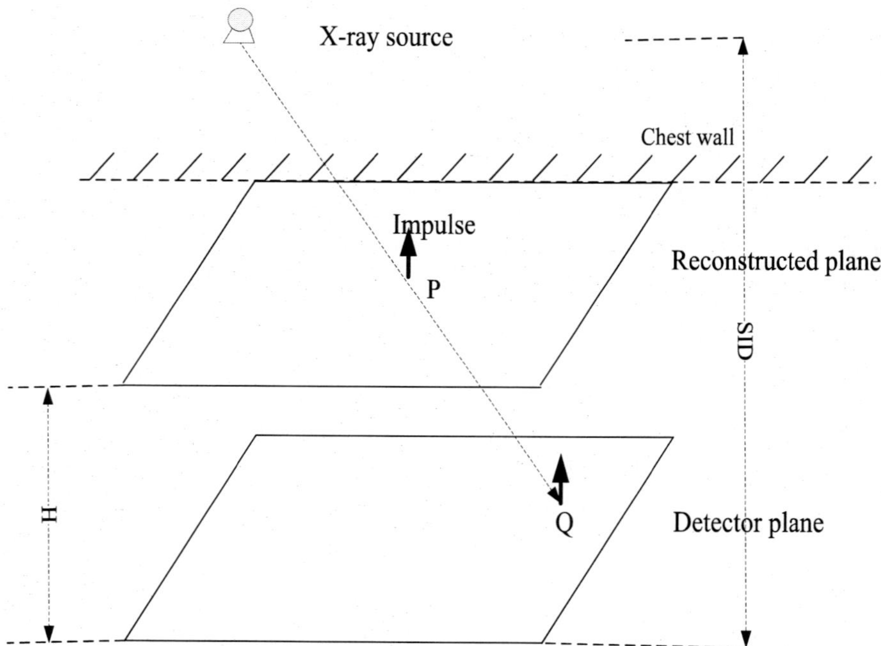

Figure 11. Impulse imaging simulation for Reconstruction MTF(f).

Figure 12 shows the MTFrecon(f) curves of BP reconstruction algorithm for the simulations with different impulse locations. Blue curves represent the MTFrecon(f) results for different impulse locations. Red curves represent the average MTFrecon(f) for the corresponding areas.

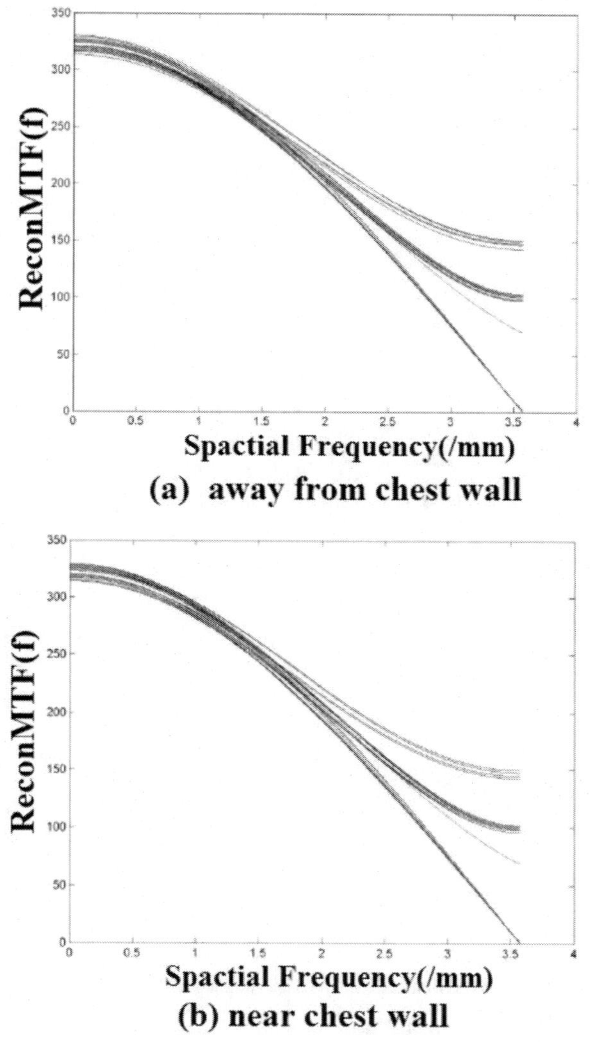

Figure 12. Reconstruction MTF(f) curves of BP in different experiments with different impulse locations. Blue curves are MTFrecon(f) of different impulses. Red curves are the average MTFrecon(f).

5.2. Noise Power Spectrum (NPS)

The *NPS(f)* is one of the most common metrics characterizing the noise property of imaging systems. The frequency-dependent *NPS(f)* is defined as the variance per frequency bin of a stochastic signal in the spatial frequency domain (Dobbins 2000). It can be directly computed from the squared Fourier amplitude of 2D imaging data by:

$$NPS(w_x, w_y) = \lim_{M,N \to \infty} (MN\Delta X\Delta Y) < \left| FT[I(x,y) - \bar{I}]\right|^2 >$$

$$= \lim_{M,N \to \infty} \lim_{K \to \infty} \frac{MN\Delta X\Delta Y}{K} \sum_{k=1}^{K} \left| FT[I(x,y) - \bar{I}]\right|^2$$

$$= \lim_{M,N,K \to \infty} \frac{\Delta X\Delta Y}{K.MN} \sum_{k=1}^{K} \left| \sum_{i=1}^{M} \sum_{j=1}^{N} [I(x_i, y_j) - \bar{I}] e^{-2\pi i(w_x x_i + w_y y_j)} \right|^2$$

(Eq. 19)

where $I(x_i, y_i)$ is the image intensity at the pixel location (x_i, y_i). $\bar{I}$ is the global mean intensity. w_x and w_y are the spatial frequencies conjugates to x and y axes. M and N are the numbers of pixels in x and y directions of the digital image. ΔX and ΔY are the pixel spacing in x and y directions, and K is the number of ROIs used for analysis.

In the experiments, a phantom, 40 mm thick, was placed on the surface of the detector. For each reconstruction algorithm, all the slice images with 1 mm slice thickness were reconstructed to cover the entire breast phantom.

In NPS calculation, regions of interest (ROIs) with the size of 1024*1024 pixels were cut from the reconstructed planes with the same height above the detector. Each ROI was evenly divided into 8 blocks with a size of 128×128 pixels. For each block, a line curve fitting through the ensemble-averaged NPS estimate was used to obtain an approximation to the greatest slope of the true NPS. Finally, the frequency components were extracted from each block and formed the smoothed NPS curves. Figure 13 illustrates the NPS curves of BP reconstruction algorithm by ten experiments. Blue curves are results of the ten experiments. The red curve is the average result.

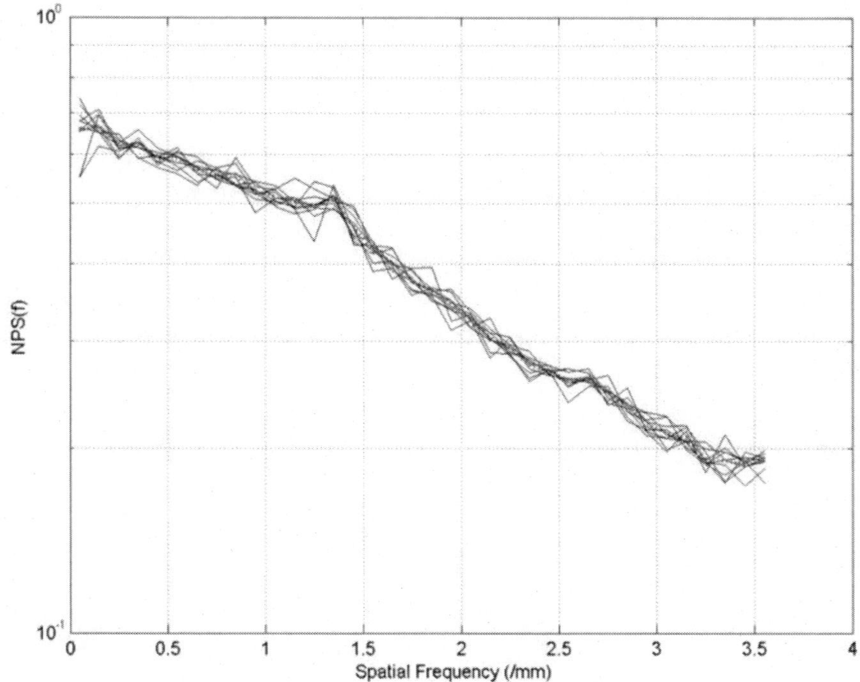

Figure 13. NPS curves of BP reconstruction with the imaging configuration VA14NP15.

5.3. Noise Equivalent Quantum (NEQ)

The relative NEQ(f) combines the modulation transfer function (MTF) of signal performance and the noise power spectrum (NPS) of noise characteristics. The relative NEQ(f) can be expressed as

$$NEQ(f) = \frac{MTF^2_{proj}(f).MTF^2_{recon}(f)}{NPS(f)} \qquad \text{(Eq. 20)}$$

The *MTFrecon(f)* is the relative MTF with the specific image reconstruction algorithm and imaging configurations. The *MTFproj(f)* is the measured MTF of the imaging system. The *NPS (f)* is the mean subtracted NPS on the same reconstruction plane.

Measured MTF$_{Recon}$ (f)

Figure 14(a) illustrates normalized reconstruction MTFs of BP, MLEM, OS-MLEM and SART with the imaging configuration of VA14NP15 for simulating impulses. Based on the normalized $MTF_{Recon}(f)$ analysis, BP has the least high-frequency response. OS-MLEM has the maximal high frequency. The difference between iterative reconstruction algorithms is very small. According to the figure, OS-MLEM shows better high-frequency response.

Figure 14(b) shows reconstruction MTF curves of two FBP versions, FBP and FBP_nogaussian. The difference is that there is no Gaussian filter in FBP_nogaussian. High-frequency response was greatly compressed after using the Gaussian low-pass filter.

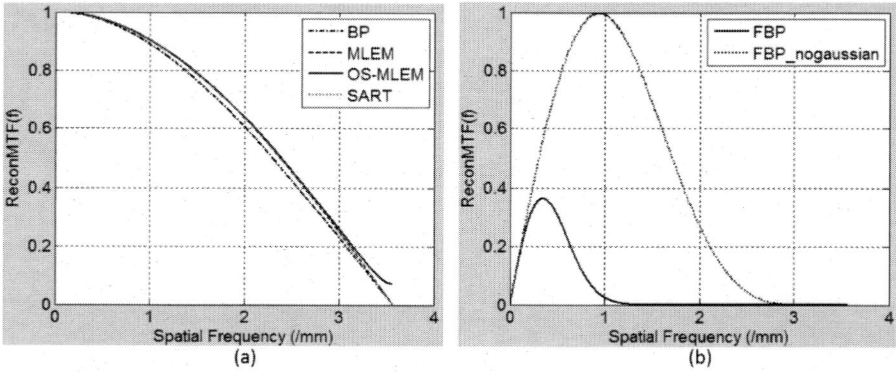

Figure14. Reconstruction MTF(f) of different reconstruction algorithms BP, MLEM, OS-MLEM and SART, (b) FBP and FBP_nogaussian.

Measured NPS(f)

Figure 15 shows the normalized mean-subtracted NPS(f) curves for BP, FBP, FBP_nogaussian, MLEM, OS-MLEM and SART. Following are the findings:

a. FBP has the high dynamic range. It has the highest low-frequency noise, but the least high frequency noise. An assumption is that in our FBP implementation, one high-pass filter and two low-pass filters were applied, including the ramp filter (a high-pass filter), Ham filter (a low-pass filter) and Gaussian filter (a low-pass filter). The two low-pass filters greatly suppresses the high-frequency noise.

b. Both OS-MLEM and SART have similar high-frequency noise. Their noise levels are higher than MLEM. Their iteration of subset-by-subset or projection-by-projection update in OS-MLEM and SART greatly speed up the convergence. The iteration has the effect of the high-pass filter, so it increases the high-frequency noise.

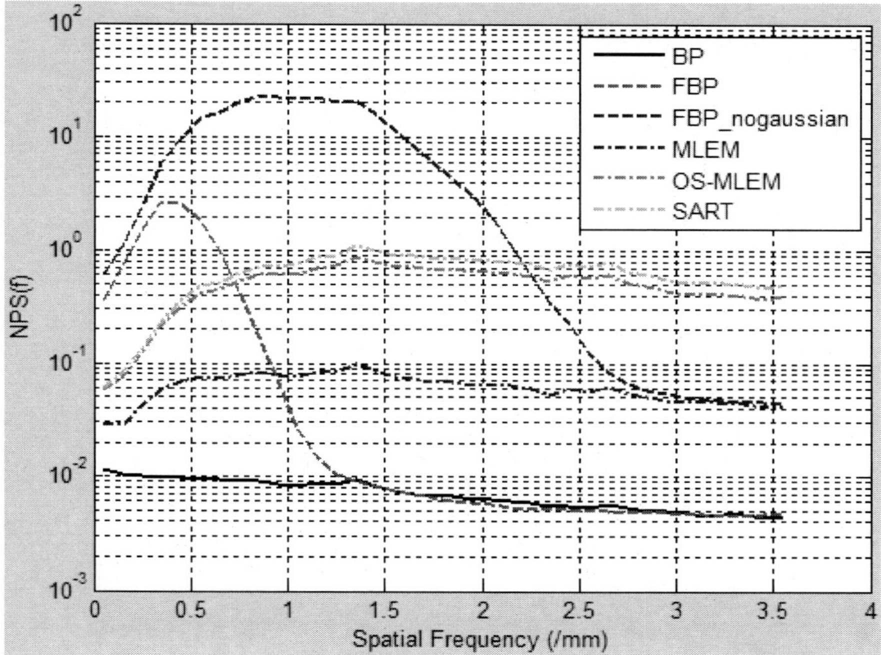

Figure 15. NPS(f) of different reconstruction algorithms.

Relative NEQ(f)

Figure 16(a) shows the relative NEQ(f) curves of MLEM, OS-MLEM and SART with the same imaging configuration VA14NP15. It suggests that MLEM has a better high-frequency response. The OS-MLEM provides a little better *NEQ(f)* response than SART. OS-MLEM is recommended in DBT reconstruction considering its overall performance, including both the image quality and computational speed.

Figure 16(b) compares the NEQ(f) of two FBP versions of FBP and FBP_nogaussian. Based on the curves, use of the Gaussian filter decreases the high-frequency response.

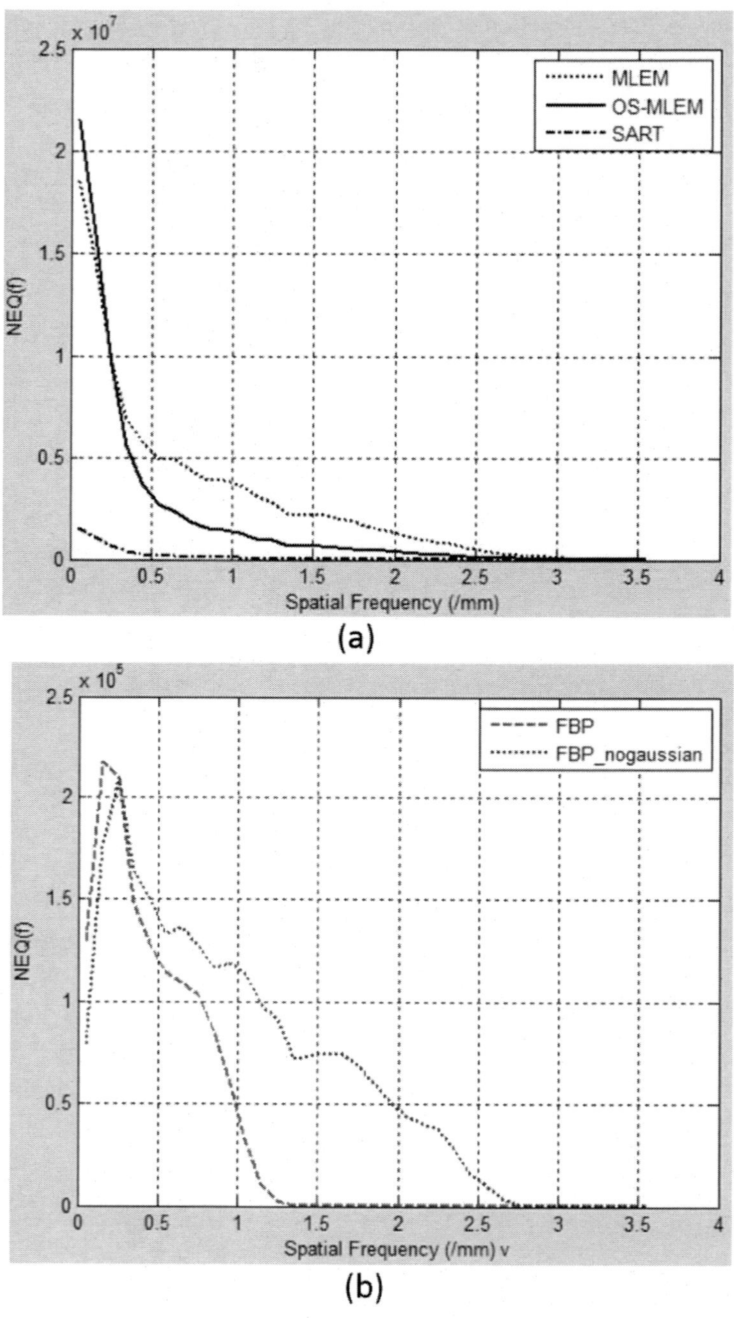

Figure 16. NEQ(f) of different reconstruction algorithms. (a) MLEM,OS_MLEM and SART, (b) FBP and FBP_nogaussian.

From the two imaging configurations, VA14NP15 and VA28NP15, tested with ten datasets of acquired NPS phantom experiments, the NEQ(f) curves of two imaging configurations in BP and FBP are intertwined. There is no obvious trend. However, in both OS-MLEM and SART, a big view angle benefits the low-frequency NEQ(f) response.

CONCLUSION

Most breast tomosynthesis systems are built upon the current digital mammography system design. The X-ray tube typically moves along an arc path above the detector. An enhanced nanotechnology enabled fast-speed multi-beam parallel breast tomosynthesis prototype system, may reduce the motion blur associated with the X-ray tubes' movement. Four methodologies were used in the optimization of image reconstruction algorithms and imaging configurations of our new system. A linear analysis method modelling the signal propagation was used to evaluate frequency characterization of blurring-out reconstruction algorithms. Computer simulations of sphere and wire were used to compare reconstruction algorithms and imaging configurations. The NEQ was investigated to evaluate reconstruction algorithms and imaging configurations in the frequency domain. According to the results, the iterative reconstruction algorithms remove more out-of-plane blur; increasing the view angle can reduce out-of-plane blur; and increasing the number of projection images can enhance the in-focus sharpness of objects.

REFERENCES

Andersen A H, Kak AC. (1984). Simultaneous algebraic reconstruction technique (SART): a new implementation of the ART algorithm. *Ultrasound Imaging*, 6: 81–94.

Andersen A H. (1989). Algebraic reconstruction in CT from limited views. *IEEE Trans. on Medical Imaging*, 8(1):50-55.

Balla A, Zhou W, Chen Y. (2010). Impulse Response Characterization of Breast Tomosynthesis Reconstruction with Parallel Imaging Configurations. *Proc. SPIE*, 76225K. 1-8.

Barrett H B, Myers K J. (2004). Foundation of Image Science. John Wiley & Sons Inc., Hoboken, New Jersey.

Chen Y, Lo J Y, Dobbins J T III. (2007a). Importance of point-by-point backprojection (BP) correction for isocentric motion in digital breast tomosynthesis: Relevance to morphology of microcalcifications. *Med. Phys.* 34(10): 3885-3892.

Chen Y, Lo J Y, Ranger N T, Samei E, Dobbins J T III. (2007b). Methodology of NEQ (f) analysis for optimization and comparison of digital breast tomosynthesis acquisition techniques and reconstruction algorithms. *Proc. SPIE;* 6510: 65101-I.

Chen Y. (2007c). Digital breast tomosynthesis (DBT) – a novel imaging technology to improve early breast cancer detection: implementation, comparison and optimization. PhD dissertation., Duke University, 2007.

Chen Y, Zhou W, Yang G, Lu J P, Zhou O. (2009). Breast tomosynthesis reconstruction with a multi-beam x-ray source. *Proc. SPIE* 7258, 725859-8(2009).

Chen Y, Balla A, Rayford CE II, Zhou W, Fang J, Cong L. (2010). Digital tomosynthesis parallel imaging computational analysis with shift and add and back projection reconstruction algorithms. *Int. J. Computational Biology and Drug Design*; 3(4): 287-296.

Cong L, Zhou W, Chen Y. (2011). Effects of slice thickness filter in filtered backprojection reconstruction with the parallel breast tomosynthesis imaging configuration. Proc. *IEEE-Int. Workshop on Genomic Signal Processing and Statistics (GENSIPS)*:194-197.

Dobbins J T III, Powell A O, Weaver Y K. (1987). Matrix inversion tomosynthesis: Initial image reconstructions. *Abstract Summaries of the RSNA*165 (P): 333.

Dobbins J T III. (1990). Matrix Inversion Tomosynthesis improvements in longitudinal x-ray slice imaging. *U.S. Patent #4,903,204.* Assignee: Duke University.

Dobbins J T III. (2000). Image quality metrics for digital systems. In *Handbook of Medical Imaging, Vol. 1. Physics and Psychophysics*, ed. J. Beutel, H. L. Kundel, and R. L. Van Metter, 161-222. SPIE.

Dobbins J T III, Godfrey D J. (2003). Digital X-ray tomosynthesis: current state of the art and clinical potential. *Phys. Med. Biol.* 48: 65-106.

Dobbins J T, Samei E, Ranger N T, Chen Y. (2006). Intercomparison of methods for image quality characterization. II. Noise power spectrum. *Med. Phys.* 33(5):1466-1475.

Erdogan H, Fessler J A. (1999). An Ordered Subsets Algorithms for Transmission Tomography, *Phys. Med. Biol.*, 44:2835.

Fujita H, Tsai D −Y, Itoh T, Doi K, Morishita J, Ueda K, Ohtsuka A. (1992). Simple Method for Determining the Modulation Transfer Function in Digital Radiography. *IEEE Trans. on Medical Imaging*; 11(1):34-39.

Godfrey D J, McAdams H P, Dobbins J T III. (2006). Optimization of the Matrix Inversion Tomosynthesis (MITS) impulse response and modulation transfer function characteristics for chest imaging. *Med. Phys.* 33(3): 655-667.

Ghosh Roy D N, Kruger R A, Yih B, Del Rio P. (1985). Selective plane removal in limited angle tomographic imaging. *Med Phys.* 12(1):65-70.

Gonzalez R C, Woods R E. (2008). Digital Image Processing. *Prentice Hall.*

Grant D G. (1972). Tomosynthesis: a three-dimensional radiographic imaging technique. *IEEE Trans. on Biomed. Eng.*, BME-19: 20-28.

Guimarães L T G, Schiabel H, Stemberg D R M. (2009). Computer Simulation in Evaluating the Attenuation Coefficients Influence on Mammography Images Contrast. *IFMBE Proc.*, 2009, Volume 25/2, 454-457, DOI: 10. 1007/978-3-642-03879-2_128.

Juliano R L, Sunnarborg S, Desimone J, Haroon Z. (2011). The Carolina Center of Cancer Nanotechnology Excellence: Past Accomplishments and Future Perspectives. *Nanomedicine* (Lond). 6(1): 19–24.

Lange K, Carson R. (1984). EM reconstruction algorithms for emission and transmission tomography. *J. Computer Assisted Tomography.* 8(2): 306-316.

Lange K, Fessler J A. (1995). Globally convergent algorithms for maximum a posteriori transmission tomography. *IEEE Trans. on Image Processing.* 4(10): 1430-1438.

Lalush D S, Quan E, Rajaram R, Zhang J, Lu J, Zhou O. (2006). Tomosynthesisreconstruction from multi-beam x-ray sources. *Proc. of IEEE Intl. Symp. on Biomedical Imaging*, 1180-1183.

Lauritsch G, Haerer W. (1998). A theoretical framework for filtered back-projection in tomosynthesis. *Proc. SPIE* 3338: 1127-1137.

Li J, Jaszczak R J, Greer K L, Coleman R E. (1993). Implementation of an accelerated iterative algorithm for cone-beam SPECT. *Phys. Med. Biol.* 39(3): 643-653.

Matsuo H, Iwata A, Horiba I, Suzumura N. (1993). Three-dimensional image reconstruction by digital tomo-synthesis using inverse filtering. *IEEE Trans. Med. Imaging* 12: 307-313.

Mertelemeier T, Orman J, Haerer W, Dudam M K. (2006). Optimizing filtered backprojection reconstruction for a breast tomosynthesis prototype device. *Proc. SPIE* 6142: 131-142.

Niklason L T, Christian B T, Niklason L E, Kopans D B, Castleberry D E, Opsahl-Ong B H, Landberg C E, Slanetz P J, Giardino A A, Moore R, Albagli D, DeJule M C, Fitzgerald P F, Fobare D F, Giambattista B W, Kwasnick R F, Liu J, Lubowski S J, Possin G E, Richotte J F, Wei C Y, Wirth R F. (1997). Digital tomosynthesis in breast imaging. *Radiology* 205:399-406.

Park J M, Franken Jr. E A, Garg M, Fajardo L L, Niklason L T. (2007). Breast tomosynthesis: present considerations and future applications. *Radiographics*. 2007;27(Suppl 1):S231-240.

Qian X, Tucker A, Gidcumb E, Shan J, Yang G, Calderon-Colon X, Sultana S, Lu J, Zhou O, Spronk D, Sprenger F, Zhang J, Kennedy D, Farbizio T, Jing Z, (2012). High Resolution Stationary Digital Breast Tomosyntheisis Using Distributed Carbon Nanotube X-Ray Source Array, *Med. Phys.* 39(4):2090-2099.

Radon J, (1917). Über die bestimmung von funktionen durch ihrd intergralwerte l ängs gewissermannigfaltigkeiten. *Ber. Verch Saechs. Akad. Wiss. Leipzig Math. Phys. Kl.* 69: 262-267.

Rayford CE II, Zhou W, Chen Y (2013). Breast tomosynthesis imaging configuration analysis. Int. *J. Computational Biol. and Drug Design*; 6:3:255-62.

Samei E, Ranger N T, Dobbins J T, Chen Y (2006). Intercomparison of methods for image quality characterization. I. Modulation transfer function. *Med. Phys.* 33(5):1454-1465.

Sprawls, P. (1998). Image Characteristics and Quality in The Physical Principles of Medical Imaging (book chapter). Medical Physics Publishing. Madison, Wisconsin.

Stevens G M, Fahrig R, Pelc N J (2001). Filtered backprojection for modifyingthe impulse response of circular tomosynthesis. *Med. Phys.* 28: 372-380.

Wu T, Stewart A, Stanton M, McCauley T, Phillips W, Kopans D B, Moore R H, Eberhard J W, Opsahl-Ong B, Niklason L, Williams M B (2003). Tomographic mammography using a limited number of low-dose cone-beam projection images. *Med. Phys.* 30: 365-380.

Wu T, Moore R H, Rafferty E A, Kopans D B (2004). A comparison of reconstruction algorithms for breast tomosynthesis. *Med. Phys.* 9: 2636-2647.

Yang G, Rajaram R, Cao G, Sultana S, Liu Z, Lalush D S, Lu J, Zhou O (2008). Stationary digital breast tomosynthesis system with a multi-beam field emission x-ray source array. *Proc. SPIE* 6913: 69131A.

Zhang Y, Chan H, Sahiner B, Wei J, Goodsitt M M, Hadjiiski L M, Ge J, Zhou C (2006). A comparative study of limited-angle cone-beam reconstruction methods for breast tomosynthesis. *Med. Phys.* 33(10): 3781-3795.

Zhou W, Balla A, Chen Y (2008). Tomosynthesis reconstruction using an accelerated expectation maximization algorithm with novel data structure based on sparse matrix ray-tracing method. *Int. J. Functional Informatics and Personalized Medicine;* 1:4: 355-365.

Zhou W, Qian X, Lu J, Zhou O, Chen Y. (2010). Multi-beam X-ray source breast tomosynthesis reconstruction with different algorithms. *Proc. SPIE* 7622H:1-8.

Zhou W (2012). Image reconstruction and imaging configuration optimization with a novel nanotechnology enabled breast tomosynthesis multi-beam X-ray system. Ph.D. dissertation Southern Illinois University Carbondale.

Zhou W, Cong L, Fang J, Qian X, Lee Y Z, Lu J, Zhou O, Chen Y. (2013). Noise power spectrum and modulation transfer function analysis of breast tomosynthesis imaging. Proc. SPIE 8868, Medical Imaging 2013: *Physics of Medical Imaging* 86684N.

Zhou W, Lu J, Zhou O, Chen Y. (2014). Evaluation of back-projection methods for breast tomosynthesis image reconstruction. *Journal of Digital Imaging;* 28(3):338-345.

Zhou W, Malalla N, Zhang Z, Chen Y. (2015a) Computer simulation and optimization of breast tomosynthesis parallel imaging configuration and reconstruction. *Int. J. Computational Biology and Drug Design*; 8(2).

Zhou W, Lu J, Zhou O, Chen Y. (2015b) Ray-tracing-based reconstruction algorithms for digital breast tomosynthesis. *J. Electron. Imaging*; 24(2) 23-28.

INDEX

clinical application, 21, 37
clinical examination, 62
clinical trials, vii, viii, 26, 27, 29, 40
clusters, 39, 46, 68, 69
competition, 73
complexity, 87, 88
composition, 6, 7
compression, 29, 33, 43, 57, 77
computed tomography, 2, 23, 33, 66
configuration, vii, viii, 75, 77, 79, 90, 92, 95, 99, 100, 101, 104, 106, 107
consensus, 51, 63
convergence, 88, 101
correlation, 42, 60
cost, 29, 31, 34, 38, 76
CT scan, 65

D

database, viii, 26, 35, 36, 72, 73, 74
death rate, viii, 25
denoising, 2, 3, 5, 21
dense breast tissues, vii, 76
deoxyribonucleic acid, 27
depth, vii, 35, 76, 90, 93
detection, viii, 2, 10, 11, 21, 22, 25, 26, 28, 30, 32, 35, 37, 38, 40, 43, 44, 45, 46, 47, 48, 49, 50, 51, 52, 53, 54, 55, 56, 57, 58, 59, 60, 62, 63, 66, 68, 76, 104
developing countries, 27
diaphysis, 19
diffraction, 28
Digital Breast Tomosynthesis, (DBT) v, vii, viii, 2, 6, 8, 9, 14, 16, 17, 21, 22, 25, 26, 27, 35, 36, 37, 38, 39, 40, 41, 42, 43, 44, 45, 46, 47, 48, 49, 50, 51, 52, 53, 54, 55, 56, 57, 58, 59, 60, 67, 68, 69, 71, 73, 74, 75, 76, 77, 78, 79, 80, 81, 82, 89, 95, 101, 104
diseases, 27
distortions, 38, 39, 44, 45
distribution, 40
DNA, 27
DOI, 105

E

enlargement, 19, 53
examinations, 23, 26, 28, 29, 30, 40, 41, 49, 53, 54, 57, 58, 62
exclusion, 5
exposure, vii, 1, 3, 5, 7, 21, 33, 79

F

false negative, 37
films, 29
filters, 84, 86, 100
fluorine, 64
Food and Drug Administration (FDA), 29, 35, 36, 37, 60, 63

G

gadolinium, 31
gamma rays, 32
geometry, 36, 66, 67, 77, 78, 84, 93
glucose, 32

H

histological examination, 57
homogeneity, 89
human, 6, 21, 71
hydrogen, 31

I

identification, 79
image analysis, 72
image interpretation, 38, 70
imaging modalities, 28, 38
imaging systems, 37, 79, 95, 97
implants, 31, 66
improvements, viii, 18, 25, 26, 28, 39, 104
impulses, 96, 97, 100
incidence, 28, 58, 60, 61

W

water, 7, 31
wavelet, 2, 3, 5, 13, 14, 15, 21
wavelet denoising, 2, 3, 21

X

x-ray tomosynthesis, vii, 22
x-ray tube angles, vii, viii, 25
x-rays, 29, 30